TABLE OF CONTENTS

Page

ACRONYMS

AAR	After Action Review
AI	Avian Influenza
CDC	Centers for Disease Control and Prevention
CI / KR	Critical Infrastructure / Key Resources
COOP	Continuity of Operations
DHS	Department of Homeland Security
EHR	Electronic Health Record
EOC	Emergency Operations Center
EOP	Emergency Operations Plan
ESAR-VHP	Emergency System for Advanced Registration of Volunteer Health Professionals
FEMA	Federal Emergency Management Agency
GAO	Government Accountability Office
HICS	Hospital Incident Command System
ICS	Incident Command System
NIMS	National Incident Management System
OSHA	Occupational Safety and Health Administration
PI	Pandemic Influenza
PPE	Personal Protective Equipment
SNS	Strategic National Stockpile
VHA	Veterans Health Administration
WHO	World Health Organization
WMD	Weapons of Mass Destruction

ILLUSTRATIONS

TABLES

CHAPTER 1

INTRODUCTION

In 1918, the world population fell victim to a pandemic –Spanish flu" claiming the lives of over 100 million people. More recently, the –Asian flu" and –Hong Kong flu," in 1957 and 1968 respectively, caused the deaths of an estimated one to four million people worldwide with each outbreak. Since the year 1580, 31 documented pandemic outbreaks have occurred, which averages to an outbreak every 12.5 years (Lazzari and Stohr 2004). The last pandemic took place 40 years ago, setting the stage for a new flu outbreak to occur at any time. Over the past decade, hospitals, public health agencies, healthcare accrediting bodies, and international organizations acknowledged the risk and created pandemic influenza preparedness plans to mitigate the next outbreak.

Current advancements in medicine enable us to treat viruses and bacterial infections, thus creating an ability to combat a pandemic influenza outbreak. However, in 1918, there was no such treatment. Therefore, if a similar event occurred today, the possibility of reducing mortality rates increases to some degree; however, it is difficult to determine how effective the medication will be against the next pandemic. For example, the current avian flu does not respond well to medications, maintaining a mortality rate greater than 60 percent with no viable vaccine. Thus, if the H5N1, avian flu were to become transmissible from person to person, the death rate could be catastrophic. Additionally, recent concerns of avian flu by researchers question whether hospitals have security plans ready to initiate, which will allow the facility to remain viable during a pandemic influenza. In this case, viable suggests the ability for a hospital to maintain its essential services, adequate staffing, and remains supplied to treat patients. Consequently, there exist concerns as to whether healthcare workers will show up to work due to fears of becoming ill or passing the illness to family members. Furthermore, incorporate into the scenario a large percentage of the US population (currently over 300,000,000), trying to access urgent healthcare, and the result is a chaos requiring security forces to maintain order. There will not be enough beds, medications, or caregivers to treat the sick. This extremely fragile situation will act as a catalyst inciting people to violence or use of force in obtaining the care or medications they feel they need. The purpose of this study is to investigate the factors ensuring hospital viability during a pandemic influenza outbreak. Subsequently, the compiled results will assist in producing a pandemic viability checklist that will aid healthcare facilities in mitigating potential threats during a pandemic influenza outbreak.

It is necessary to briefly discuss the tenants of emergency management to provide a foundation that enables the understanding of the process. First, it is important to understand the hierarchy of responsibility. Thus, the local area where the incident occurs is responsible to meet the needs of the residents and respond to the emergency. If the local area becomes overwhelmed and can no longer function, the state then assists the local area with the response and recovery. Furthermore, if the state cannot meet the needs of the incident, federal assets are then requested to meet the local needs. For the system to work properly each level of the government from local to state and to federal must have an understanding of emergency management and the roles each other bear.

Secondly, emergency management consists of four phases: mitigation, preparedness, response, and recovery. Each phase represents a period of time in relation to an incident. The mitigation phase begins after an organization performs a threat assessment or Hazard Vulnerability Analysis (HVA), which determines the most likely threats facing the facility and the estimated risk associated with the hazard. Hospitals are required to perform an HVA annually if they are accredited by the Joint Commission, which instituted this requirement in 2001 (Steinhauer and Bauer 2002). Once the threats have been determined, the organization can work to mitigate the hazards with the available resources. It is up to the administration to determine the risk level that is acceptable if funding prohibits instituting mitigation measures (The Institute for Crisis, Disaster, and Risk Management at the George Washington University; for the Veterans Health Administration /US 2006).

The preparedness phase involves formulating and planning processes and procedures, which will be in effect during the response phase. Typically, the planning culminates into the hospital's Emergency Operations Plan (EOP), which provides the ―how to" during the response and assigns personnel to act as a primary or back up in certain roles. The EOP is generally combined with or based upon the Hospital Incident Command System (HICS) and sometimes the National Incident Management System (NIMS). These systems act as frameworks to assist organizations in their planning and provide templates for role responsibilities and coordination requirements with local and state entities.

The next phase is incident response, which executes the plan produced in the preparedness phase. People and equipment are moving very quickly to meet the needs of the emergency and assist the victims affected by the incident. Most hospitals will operate with an Emergency Operations Center (EOC) during the response phase, which is the command and control center for facility operations, as well as coordination and communication with other organizations. It is important to collect as much information as possible during and following the emergency to assist in improving the future response. Many times these are called After Action Reviews (AAR), which provide evaluations, critiques, and successes of the incident response (McGlown 2004).

The last phase of emergency management is recovery, also called continuity of operations (COOP). Unfortunately, this seems to be the phase that organizations spend the least time planning. A good recovery or continuity plan will ensure a hospital does not have to close its doors, even if the building receives damage from an existing threat, such as a hurricane or manmade terrorist event. During this phase, healthcare facilities should have an agreement with at least one, if not two organizations for an alternate temporary hospital site. Possible sites include churches with large cultural halls or gymnasiums with an adequate power and water supply. The bottom line is that the recovery should focus on restoring the essential services, such as power, water, and sewer. Additionally, this should be occurring at the same time as the response phase, or as soon as possible depending on the situation (Steinhauer and Bauer 2002). The phases of emergency management act as a cycle of continual improvement and assist the hospital to remain viable during incidents.

Most hospital functions continue during all phases of emergency management, which creates a challenging environment in the event of an incident. An essential element that cannot be overlooked during emergency management operations is security. Hospital security is important during a pandemic due to large numbers of patients trying to access a limited amount of resources, which may lead to frustration and violence. Another factor of security is providing a safe environment for the healthcare workers to function, thus

4

promoting the staff to attend work during an emergency. Additionally, security is necessary within the hospital to guard patient information, medications, vaccinations, limited supplies, and patient safety.

Consequently, logistics security for pharmaceuticals and other various supplies will be of paramount importance. Initially, the primary way to treat the pandemic flu will be through antiviral medications such as ―Tamiflu.‖ Many will grow increasingly ill and develop pneumonia, which is usually treated with antibiotics. A vaccine will not be available for several months, thus any stocks of these medications will deplete rapidly. Consequently, pharmacies in and out of the hospital will be a prime target for theft, looting, and civil unrest. Security requirements, in and out of the hospital will demand additional assistance, either from the military or private security firms hired by businesses to protect their assets. These security issues rarely receive consideration in emergency management plans, but can be the key to ensure healthcare facilities remain viable during a pandemic outbreak.

Primary Research Question

Understanding the emergency management process is the beginning to uncovering actions the healthcare industry should undertake during catastrophes. However, the ―all hazards‖ approach is inadequate to respond to a moderate pandemic outbreak. Shortcomings of our fragile healthcare framework combined with the prolonged duration of a pandemic make it difficult to prepare for such a catastrophic disaster. Therefore, the purpose of this study is to determine, what should hospitals do to remain viable during a pandemic influenza outbreak?

Secondary Research Questions

To answer the primary research question, the following secondary questions should be addressed: Should either the military or private security be utilized to augment security at hospitals? What should hospitals do to encourage their employees to show up for work during an outbreak of Pandemic Influenza? What are the significant aspects of hospital security during a pandemic influenza outbreak? These questions are all significant, but the most important is the ability for a hospital to remain viable during a pandemic. Subsequently, it is difficult for a hospital to remain viable without addressing these secondary research questions. Thus, their importance exists as building blocks to determine how a hospital can continue to keep its doors open during the largest and longest mass casualty event of most healthcare workers' careers.

To answer these questions it will be necessary to provide a history of pandemic influenza and introduce current findings on how to mitigate the threat. Additionally, a comparative case study will be utilized to determine common measures that will assist the hospital in remaining viable during the event. The accumulation of the hospital viability measures coupled with its subsequent analysis will be the basis for answering the study's questions and providing guidance to the healthcare industry today.

CHAPTER 2

LITERATURE REVIEW

A pandemic influenza outbreak is a real threat to the United States and its citizens. Only planning and preparation will assist in mitigating the effects of such a potentially devastating occurrence. The purpose of this section is to present historical case studies and provide current information about pandemic influenza (PI) planning, which relates to the study's research questions. Understanding these topics will assist in the fusion of salient points with findings from the case studies to answer the primary research question and generate a hospital viability checklist for a PI incident to utilize as a guide ensuring the safety of patients and employees.

Historical Case Studies

Many lessons can be learned from history, especially when investigating similar occurrences. In the past century, there were several cases, which have relevance when discussing pandemic influenza: 1918 Spanish Flu, 1957 Asian Flu, 1968 Hong Kong Flu, 2003 SARS epidemic, and 2005 Hurricane Katrina. Understanding the background of each of these cases will provide insight about these disasters and possible techniques to mitigate their impact on society.

In 1918, as the United States was involved in World War I, a new influenza virus was emerging somewhere in America that would eventually spread worldwide and kill somewhere between 50 to 100 million people (Barry 2005). The transmission occurred along lasting pioneer trails and trade routes. Additionally, as the troops traveled to Europe, they took the virus with them assisting in its eventual pandemic route. The

Spanish Flu had three waves, which lasted the better part of two years and devastated the US economy (Garrett 2008). This case provides numerous accounts and lessons learned making it ideal to provide answers to this study's research questions.

Another case was the 1957 Asian Flu, which is believed to have begun near Hong Kong involving over 250,000 people in a short time span. Samples of the virus arrived in Washington DC, at Walter Reed Army Medical Center where it was analyzed. Subsequently, a vaccine was developed and for the first time a mass vaccination occurred (Kilbourne 2006). This virus was different from the 1918 Spanish Flu as it was a reassortment of two influenza viruses, meaning two viruses merged to form a new virus (Garcia-Sastre and Whitley 2006). Similar to the 1918 Flu, the pandemic made several waves and lasted for two years killing between one to four million worldwide (World Health Organization 2009). The 1957 Asian Flu was much milder than the 1918 Spanish Flu and has not had the same amount of focus or lessons learned produced to make this a useful case for this study, but has relevance as a major pandemic in the last century.

Additionally, the 1968 Hong Kong Flu serves an important case in history. Similarly to the 1957 Asian Flu, it had its roots in Asia, emerged through reassortment, and killed between one and four million worldwide in a two year period (Belshe 2005). The most interesting thing about the pandemic is this Type A influenza virus (H3N2) or its variants are still responsible for most of the annual influenza strains since 1968 (Davenport 2008). Even though, the Hong Kong Flu is interesting and still deserves respect today, it does not have numerous sources of historical reference to be supportive as a case study in this thesis.

More recently, in 2003 emerged a new coronavirus called severe acute respiratory syndrome (SARS) originating in the Guandong Province of China. A physician from the Guandong Province visited Hong Kong and infected several others at the hotel he stayed at; then they carried it to Vietnam, Canada, and Singapore. In just over two months, the number of cases grew to 8,459 cases with 805 deaths, resulting in almost a 10 percent mortality rate (Engman 2002). It is the belief that global surveillance coupled with intense public health measures controlled the spread of SARS and eventually stopped the transmission of the disease (Svoboda et al. 2004). This is an especially interesting case due to the high mortality rate associated with SARS, advanced emergency management practices, and the successful control of the disease. For these reasons, SARS makes an excellent case study from which to answer the studies research questions.

Another historical case occurred in 2005; Hurricane Katrina devastated the Gulf Coast region affecting multiple states and over a half million people. Hurricane Katrina caused catastrophic damage to some areas in the region resulting in one of the largest relief efforts in US history (GAO 2005). Ultimately, the storm killed more than 1,300 people and uncovered multiple flaws in the existing emergency management process between local, State, and Federal response (Department of Defense 2006). Although this is not specifically an influenza case, it provides multiple lessons learned about a regional disaster that crippled all levels of response and exposed significant shortcomings in preparedness making it a good case study to utilize in this project.

These cases present focused material to study and analyze the measures, which will enable hospitals to remain viable during a catastrophic incident such as a moderate to severe pandemic. The lessons learned from these cases will add to the future measures that will assist in preparing for possible disasters. It is imperative to learn from past mistakes to ensure they are not made again. Thus, the combination of information from past case studies and current plans or procedures will provide comprehensive measures to mitigate future threats.

<u>Pandemic Influenza Planning</u>

In the past decade, PI has become a premier topic among emergency managers due to the increasing occurrence of avian influenza outbreaks in China and throughout Asia coupled with similar concerns of biological weapons of mass destruction (WMD). These concerns have created interest globally resulting in pandemic planning nationally and filtering down to state and local governments. However, these governments must rely on many private organizations, such as hospitals, to assist in the event of a pandemic flu. The difficulty that exists in relying on private organizations is that many are commercial businesses and they must remain profitable. Subsequently, emergency response preparedness is a significant investment by private organizations and must balance efficiency with meeting emergency management standards within the industry. If the private organizations are unable to respond to a pandemic, the federal government will incur the responsibility to provide relief in the form of money and personnel to augment the most affected areas. Consequently, current planning is insufficient in meeting the needs of the public. In order to effectively present pandemic influenza planning the following elements will be discussed:

1. National Policies
2. Avian Influenza

3. Strategic National Stockpile

4. Vaccinations

5. Biological Warfare

6. Mitigation Techniques

7. Hospital Viability

8. Domestic Security

These elements of pandemic planning will serve to broadly enhance individuals understanding of the current processes and will provide insight as to the need for this comparative case study.

National Policies

National policies serve as a framework and guide to the states and local areas to assist in developing their own emergency management or disaster plans. Several of the policies and plans include the Incident Command System (ICS), the National Incident Management System (NIMS), the Hospital Incident Command System (HICS), the National Strategy for Pandemic Influenza Implementation Plan, and The Pandemic Influenza, Preparedness, Response, and Recovery Guide for Critical Infrastructure and Key Resources. These resources are free of charge and can be readily accessed on the internet, thus providing a place for organizations to start their own planning.

The ICS has been integrated into the NIMS, which was developed in accordance from presidential directive HSPD-5 in 2003 stating,

> The Secretary shall develop, submit for review to the Homeland Security Council, and administer a National Incident Management System (NIMS). This system will provide a consistent nationwide approach for Federal, State, and local governments to work effectively and efficiently together to prepare for, respond to, and recover from domestic incidents, regardless of cause, size, or complexity.

11

To provide for interoperability and compatibility among Federal, State, and local capabilities, the NIMS will include a core set of concepts, principles, terminology, and technologies covering the incident command system. (Bush 2003, 2-3)

NIMS provides a foundation for first responders in reaction to natural disasters, terrorist attacks, and other emergencies. In addition, all federal agencies are mandated to implement NIMS, while funding to states and local agencies are tied to its use (U.S. Department of Homeland Security 2004). Similarly, HICS provides healthcare facilities with industry specific adaptations from ICS and is consistent with NIMS by implementing the 17 elements of the hospital-based guidelines (CA Emergency Medical Services Authority 2006). These resources serve to provide an ‑All-Hazards" response capability to the organizations and agencies implementing their guidance.

NIMS and HICS are not specific enough for some disasters, such as Pandemic Influenza. Therefore, DHS has provided the National Strategy for Pandemic Influenza Implementation Plan, which offers general guidance for international cooperation, federal government response, law enforcement, and the protection of human health (U.S. Department of Homeland Security 2006). Additionally, The Pandemic Influenza, Preparedness, Response, and Recovery Guide for Critical Infrastructure and Key Resources offer the private sector guidelines to follow during a pandemic outbreak. It is vitally important that public and private sector take the threat of pandemic influenza seriously as warned by Department of Homeland Security (DHS) Secretary Michael Chertoff stating, ‑The avian flu bears the potential for societal disruption of unprecedented proportion. Strong partnerships and smart planning will be our best protection against this threat" (U.S. Department of Homeland Security 2006, 4). Traditional emergency management lacks the ability to adequately respond to the global threat of pandemic influenza. Therefore, a pandemic requires special attention by all entities to overcome the awesome response needed during such a disaster. These emergency management systems and guides will work to alleviate a portion of the need if implemented by the key agencies responsible for essential services. Additionally, understanding how these plans relate provides insight how a hospital will operate during a pandemic and how they can request assistance from governmental agencies.

Avian Influenza

Understanding Avian Influenza (AI) is crucial in the mitigation of its effects on humanity. However, prior to discussing AI it is beneficial to describe human influenza and its effects on society. The influenza virus, characterized as the seasonal flu, is easily spread through large droplets of fluid from the nose or mouth of infected persons, which is produced when they sneeze or cough. Additionally, infection can occur when persons are exposed to objects that are contaminated by touch or aerosolized infected droplets (OSHA 2007). The influenza virus infects the upper respiratory tract of humans, which can cause pneumonia. This viral version of pneumonia may be fatal and usually occurs in the pediatric and geriatric populations. Subsequent bacterial infections may also occur from the influenza virus, which too can cause death. Each year the average mortality rate due to complications from influenza is between 3,000 and 20,000 deaths (U.S. Department of Defense 2004). The seasonal flu remains a significant health risk, but is relatively inconsequential when compared to the lethality of AI.

Avian influenza is not a new thing; however, what concerns experts are that all of the pandemics in the past century came from avian influenza strains. Thus, during the three previous pandemics, the avian flu virus mutated into a strain that was

13

communicated between people and not just bird to human contact (Thompson and Van Gorder 2007). Two types of avian influenza exist, low pathogenic AI and highly pathogenic AI. Low pathogenic AI is transferred from wild to domesticated poultry and the symptoms are usually light or nonexistent, bearing almost no threat to humans. In contrast, highly pathogenic AI, also transferred from wild to domestic poultry, is usually deadly. This current, more deadly virus is also known as H5N1 avian influenza, or bird flu. In the past several years, the bird flu has infected over 200 people, who primarily had extensive contact with infected poultry (US Department of Health and Human Services n.d.). Unfortunately, this strain of influenza has a case fatality rate of over 50 percent, which is a frightening disclosure (Nuno et al. 2008). Additionally, current estimates suggest that approximately one third of the population in the United States would become ill and nearly two million American citizens would die (Thompson and Van Gorder 2007). This estimate may be extremely conservative with a fatality rate of 50 percent, which suggests it is similar to the deadly pandemic in 1918 that claimed upwards of 100 million worldwide (Tabery and Mackett III 2008). Consequently, it is very important to gain an understanding of AI and its potential to disrupt life, in order to determine how a hospital can mitigate its effects if it becomes a pandemic.

National Stockpile

One of the largest mitigation efforts in response to AI is the Strategic National Stockpile (SNS). ―The SNS is a federally-maintained cache of pharmaceuticals and other medical supplies that can be deployed to any location in the nation in response to a terrorist attack or other public health emergency" (Association of State and Territorial Health Officials 2008, 1). The idea for a national stockpile rests with the ability to treat

14

viral infections and other various illnesses. Treating viruses is a relatively recent breakthrough in our healthcare capabilities, which provides us with some sort of weapon against pandemic influenza that we have previously not had. "The use of antiviral medication for *short-term prophylaxis* of household contacts of a suspected or confirmed case of influenza (post exposure prophylaxis) during the very early stages of a pandemic may assist in reducing transmission of infection" (Indiana State Department of Health 2006, 32). Thus, the ability to reduce the transmission rate, as well as, the mortality rate, will lessen the overall effect on the United States as a whole.

Current estimates maintain that one third of the U.S population will become ill. Consequently, the federal government plans to stockpile approximately 100 million doses of antiviral medications through the SNS and other state stockpiles (U.S. Department of Homeland Security 2006). These stockpiles will be pushed to affected outbreak areas for local health departments and healthcare facilities to utilize in the treatment of the ill. Armed with the SNS, the federal government is positioning the United States as the leader amongst the nations of the world in the fight against pandemic influenza. Conversely, the SNS should not be seen as the "Trojan Horse" allowing the private sector and citizens to do nothing in the preparation for a pandemic event as efficacy of the medications may be unreliable in response to the new virus. The ability to overcome such an event will require everyone to take upon themselves responsibilities to reduce the effects of PI. Thus, hospitals should consider the SNS as a supplement to their own efforts in pandemic preparedness.

Vaccinations

Vaccinations are an important weapon in the defense of human disease. Thus, it is important to understand the factors surrounding the use of vaccines during a pandemic. A vaccine that is effective in protecting humans against the H5N1 AI virus would be the best alternative to reduce the effects of a pandemic if caused by that particular avian strain. Unfortunately, we do not know which virus will cause the next pandemic, but we do know that the last three pandemics occurred from influenza type A, that occurs in both birds and humans. The great concern is that the H5N1virus will mutate enabling the transmission of the virus from human to human; whereas, the current transmission of the virus is from bird to human transmission. Since the discovery of the H5N1 virus in 1997, there have been over 300 confirmed cases in many countries around the world. It is from these cases an H5N1 vaccine has been developed. Unfortunately, the current vaccine is insufficiently immunogenic and poorly matches the principal occurring strain (Toner et al. 2006).

Conversely, one of the trial vaccines showing promise requires two very large doses of the vaccine, approximately six times the normal influenza dose. The main concern with this vaccine is the sheer volume required to immunize persons, which suggests hundreds of millions of doses are needed to combat a pandemic. Another concern with producing a vaccine is the inability to know which strain variant will mutate causing the pandemic. Even with several trial vaccines, it will be difficult to know whether the initial vaccine will provide enough protection to reduce morbidity during the first wave of the pandemic. Additionally, it is unknown whether the vaccine would produce subclinical infections causing the host to become asymptomatic (Haque, Hober and Kaspert 2007). This could exacerbate transmission around the globe by creating a modern day ―Typhoid Mary." Furthermore, vaccines are generally manufactured using eggs, thus increasing the risk to individuals who are allergic to eggs becoming more susceptible to adverse reactions from the vaccine (U.S. Department of Defense 2004).

Another factor surrounding the use of vaccines to combat PI is the length of time it will take to produce the vaccine for widespread immunization. The approximate time from virus identification to the development of a vaccine is six months and several more to manufacture it for distribution, which will make it unavailable for the first wave of the pandemic (Schoch-Spana 2000). It is during the gap in this timeline, which will prove most deadly to the world's population. ―The ‗Gap‘ is the time between the first efficient human to human transmission of the virus and the availability of the vaccine to the public 9 to 12 months later" (Thompson and Van Gorder 2007, 89). Subsequently, making any advances to the current vaccine prior to the pandemic will prove invaluable during the gap to slow transmission throughout the first two waves of the pandemic. Thus, hospitals will need to plan how they will remain viable during the gap until the vaccine is ready for mass inoculation.

Bioterrorism

Similar to PI, bioterrorism provides many of the same challenges, while revealing one main difference. Bioterrorism is defined as ―the intentional release of potentially deadly germs to harm people," (Glabman 2001, 30) while PI occurs naturally. The intentional release may be a naturally occurring disease such as smallpox, or it may be a genetically engineered virus with no known cure. Whatever the case, bioterrorism is a frightening prospect, which should be considered as dangerous as PI. Additionally, bioterrorism is sometimes confused with chemical warfare. The difference between bioterrorism and chemical warfare is that bioterrorism is differentiated by a slow onset of symptoms rather than an immediate response. Issues surrounding a bioterror attack may include the outbreak itself, which will first be noted in emergency departments close to the epicenter, civil disobedience due to the lack of adequate medical care, and defection of healthcare workers for fear of contagion (Glabman 2001). Undoubtedly, a bioterror event would quickly overwhelm a hospitals capacity to treat patients, which will require vast human resources, equipment, and supplies.

The Joint Commission, a worldwide healthcare accrediting agency, requires participating hospitals to maintain an "all-hazards" approach pertaining to emergency response. However, there is anxiety that the requirements are not adequate to address a bioterrorism event, much less a pandemic (Henning et al. 2004). In 2003, a GAO report to Congress suggests many hospitals lack surge capacity and equipment to respond to a bioterror event (See Table 1). Additionally, the GAO advocates the need to be better prepared for such an event, but realizes the expenses required to purchase additional equipment and prepare to surge personnel when these costly commodities are only needed during a disaster (GAO 2003). Furthermore, skepticism exists whether hospitals should specifically plan for a bioterrorist event due to the limited resources available during such a catastrophe; however, the consensus is that performing regular tabletop exercises in response to a bioterrorism event or PI is a vital factor to overall emergency preparedness (Henning et al. 2004). Consequently, the close relationship between bioterrorism and PI provide the ability to make general preparations, which will benefit a hospitals ability to remain viable in the response to either disaster.

18

Table 1.   U.S. Hospital Capability

2 to lot	
5 to les	
10 or n	
Total per	
Number c	
Less th	
2 to les	
5 to les	
10 or m	
Total perc	

Source: GAO, ―Hospital Preparedness: Most Urban Hospital Have Emergency Plans but Lack Certain Capacities for Bioterrorism Response." 2003, 15, Table 2.

Mitigation Across Public/Private Sector

Similarly, just as general preparations for bioterrorism and PI are important in reducing the disaster's effects, so is the ability to mitigate them when they occur. Thus, in order to provide a broad picture of PI, it is vitally important to explain current techniques for mitigating the probable effects of such a widespread disaster. Mitigation of PI should occur within all levels of government, community, healthcare facilities, and even by families. It will require the collaborative effort to decrease the damage of critical infrastructure and key resources (CI/KR's) associated during a pandemic.

Critical infrastructure and key resources (See figure 1) as stated by the U.S. government (U.S. Department of Homeland Security 2006) includes:

Critical Infrastructure

1. Food and Agriculture

2. National Monuments and Icons

3. Banking and Finance

4. Chemical and Hazardous Materials

5. Defense Industrial Base

6. Water

7. Public Health and Healthcare

8. Energy

9. Emergency Services

10. Information Technology

11. Telecommunications

12. Postal and Shipping

13. Transportation

Key Resources

1. Government Facilities

2. Dams

3. Commercial Facilities

4. Nuclear Power Plants

These CI/KR's are vitally important to the stability of the United States because they act as the lifeblood to our modern society. Simple services such as water, power, gas, public transportation, and grocery stores, which many Americans take for granted, may be disrupted due to employees not showing up for work because of illness or fear of becoming sick. If a prolonged pandemic disrupts these essential systems, then public unrest is sure to follow.

Figure 1.   17 National Critical Infrastructure and Key Resources
Source: U.S. Department of Homeland Security, ―Pandemic Influenza, Preparedness, Response, and Recovery Guide for Critical Infrastructure and Key Resources," September 19, 2006, 7.

It is for this reason mitigation measures should focus on the CI/KRs. However, it is not the intention of this paper to discuss the specifics of each CI/KR in relation to mitigating the effects of a disaster, but to provide a general overview of various mitigation concepts designed to lessen the overall impact of the pandemic. Consequently, to discuss the mitigation concepts it is necessary to elaborate how the following entities view mitigation: government, businesses, individuals and hospitals. Each entity will have a different focus, but all will have the goal of remaining viable during a pandemic.

When the next pandemic arrives, the Federal Government will be expected to provide answers, direction, and assistance to the American people to ultimately decrease mortality rates in the country. No matter what preparations the federal, state, and local governments have made, the American citizens will cry that it is not enough. This is evident by the recent hurricanes, Rita and Katrina. Many thought the government did not do enough in a timely manner for those affected. Additionally, these disasters were a regional problem that allowed other areas of the country and the world to provide assistance to the gulf region. Conversely, in the event of a pandemic, the illness will spread quickly across the entire country and outside assistance seen in previous disasters will not be present.

In reaction to the disjointed response of Hurricane Katrina, the Federal Government re-evaluated the national response plan and the responsibilities of each level of the government from local to state and state to federal to ensure these failures would not happen again. The result was an overhaul of the Federal Emergency Management Agency (FEMA), which placed them subordinate to the Department of Homeland Security (DHS). FEMA still responds to disasters, but now has the added benefit of DHS resources to assist them. Moreover, the Federal Government does not have to wait for a request from the state or states to assist, but can begin making response preparations at the time of disaster or in many cases pre-positioning assets for a faster response. Restructuring the national response capabilities enables future mitigation of disasters through providing more resources than FEMA previously held.

Additionally, the Federal Government recommends state and local governments create and maintain a comprehensive emergency management plan, which provides an all-hazards approach ranging from terrorism to natural disasters. Since PI has the potential to cause such widespread turmoil, each state and local government should develop a specific PI plan. It is imperative that the local governments plan to respond without the Federal Government because they will be unable to provide assistance in the same manner as a natural disaster due to the widespread effects of the pandemic (U.S. Department of Homeland Security 2006). Thus, it is the responsibility of private business organizations and local government to create specific response measures for their area while the Federal Government is working on general mitigation measures for the Country.

Furthermore, the Department of Homeland Security outlines the role of the Federal Government in the National Strategy for Pandemic Influenza Implementation plan is as follows (U.S. Department of Homeland Security 2006):

Three Pillars for PI Strategy

1. Preparedness and communication

2. Surveillance and detection

3. Response and containment

Goals of the Federal Response

1. Stop, slow, or otherwise limit the spread of a pandemic to the United States

2. Limit the domestic spread of a pandemic, and mitigate disease, suffering and death

3. Sustain infrastructure and mitigate impact to the economy and the functioning of society

Federal Government Primary Responsibilities

1. The support of containment efforts overseas and limitation of the arrival of a pandemic to our shores

2. Guidance related to protective measures that should be taken

3. Modifications to the law and regulations to facilitate the national pandemic response

4. Modifications to monetary policy to mitigate the economic impact of a pandemic on communities and the nation

5. Procurement and distribution of vaccine and antiviral medications

6. Acceleration of research and development of vaccines and therapies during the outbreak

7. Federal Government Actions to Implement the National Strategy for PI

International Efforts

1. Establish surveillance capability in countries at risk

2. Expand capacity for animal health activities and press for a strong international leadership role

3. Support a coordinated response by the international community in support of national efforts

4. Coordinate public communication

5. Assist U.S. citizens traveling or living abroad

Transportation and Borders

1. Modeling to inform transportation and border decisions

2. Screening mechanisms and travel restrictions

3. Quarantine and isolation of travelers

4. Trade and movement of cargo

5. Sustaining the transportation infrastructure

Protecting Human Health

1. Achieving national goals for production and stockpiling of vaccine and antiviral medications

2. Prioritizing and distributing limited supplies of vaccine and antiviral medications

3. Deploying limited federal assets and resources to support local medical surge

4. Establishing real-time clinical surveillance

5. Modeling to inform decision making and public health interventions

Protecting Animal Health

1. Bolstering domestic surveillance

2. Expanding the national veterinary stockpile

3. Educating bird owners

4. Advancing our domestic outbreak response plans

5. Enhancing infrastructure for animal health research and development

Law Enforcement, Public Safety, and Security

1. Providing guidance to state and local law enforcement entities

2. Supporting local law enforcement activities

In summary, this outline provides a framework for the Federal Government to plan for and provide actions to mitigate a pandemic occurrence. Any concerns beyond these listed are the responsibility of states, local government, private business, communities, and individuals. Each topic of the outline deserves adequate description and explanation; however, only the relevant points to this study will be discussed further.

Ultimately, the Federal Government may quarantine certain areas in the United States and limit travel in, out, and throughout the country. This task will require activation of the National Guard and possibly federal security assets to assist with augmentation. Additionally, civil unrest could occur in areas without adequate healthcare capacity or limited essential resources. If the local law enforcement agencies are unable to take action or need assistance, federal assets will likely respond to deal with the situation. Of course, this will be predicated upon how widespread the pandemic is and the amount of federal resources available. As previously discussed, the federally held SNS will be distributed for treatment of infected persons and for prophylaxis of key personnel to utilize as a preventative measure allowing CI/KR to remain operational (U.S. Department of Health Affairs 2006). This will occur in cooperation with state government, local public health agencies, hospitals, National Guard assets, and other federal agencies. These actions by the Federal Government are designed to mitigate the spread and limit the affects of a pandemic. Thus, understanding the role of the Federal, State, and local governments in a pandemic provides insight as to what the local hospital should do in preparation for an outbreak.

Just as various forms of government must plan to mitigate a pandemic, so must private businesses in the community. Unfortunately, many businesses do not have the resources or funds to prepare for a pandemic flu. Private businesses are struggling to keep their companies profitable; nonetheless, following the current plan, we will rely on private corporations to plan to support the greater population with whatever services they provide during this tragic period. Initially, expect confusion and fear followed by ingenuity in overcoming barriers to gradually adapt and prosper in the austere pandemic environment. Those businesses who fail to plan or adapt quickly, simply will not survive. Communities must pull together and form collaborative partnerships that will work together to respond to a pandemic and other disasters.

Thus, in order for a business to endure the pandemic several basic guidelines exist in developing a business continuity plan. During a pandemic, the Occupational Safety and Health Administration (OSHA) suggests implementing protection measures such as modifying work practices, engineering controls, administrative controls, and personal protective equipment (PPE). The following are examples of each protection measure (OSHA 2007):

Work Practices

1. Providing work environment promoting personal hygiene to include the use of tissues, hand sanitizer, hand soap, paper towels, no-touch trash cans, and disinfectants

2. Encouraging employees to obtain an annual influenza vaccine

3. Provide education and training about influenza

4. Develop policies or procedures to limit contact between fellow employees and customers

Engineering Control

1. Installing physical barriers, such as clear plastic sneeze guards

2. Installing a drive-through window for customer service

3. Creating negative pressure hospital rooms

Administrative controls

1. Implement policies encouraging ill personnel to stay at home without fear of reprisals

2. Limit unnecessary travel

3. Consider teleconferences, email, flexible work hours, working from home, etc. to limit face to face contact with employees

4. Consider home delivery of your goods and services to limit the customers need to visit your workplace

5. Develop emergency communications plan between employees

Personal Protective Equipment (PPE)

1. Selected based upon the hazard to the employee

2. Properly fitted and some must be periodically refitted

3. Conscientiously and properly worn

4. Regularly maintained and replaced as necessary

5. Properly removed and disposed of to avoid contamination of self, others, or the environment

These protection measures serve as guidelines for businesses to contemplate as they address risks associated with their specific industry. Furthermore, it is vitally important for those industries on the CI/KR list to develop business continuity plans to ensure the economic and political stability of our nation.

Industries of specific importance include the transportation industry, grocery industry, and healthcare industry. The healthcare industry will be covered in detail later in the chapter precluding its necessity in this section. Moreover, these industries require the most employee to customer or patient contact than any others from the CI/KR list. The transportation industry to include rail, shipping, and trucking services provide a vital role in our modern economy. Individuals are no longer self-sufficient, but are dependent upon commodities tied to a global economy. Consequently, because transportation networks link economies, provide critical infrastructures with working material, and supply citizens with necessary commodities, disrupted transportation systems can lead to cascading failures in social and economic systems" (Luke and Rodrigue 2008, 99). Subsequently, if consumers want the necessities available in stores, then we need to ensure the safety of the individuals working in the transportation industry as well as the grocery industry.

Providing a safe environment will not be easy, but the implementation of engineering and administrative controls, as suggested earlier will assist in this endeavor. Additionally, providing employees with PPE coupled with strict personal hygiene measures will alleviate much of the threat. Moreover, it will be necessary to provide prophylaxis of antiviral's such as Tamiflu to employees in this industry just as it is planned for the healthcare industry. The grocery industry will need to make some changes in work practices to reduce the contact between people. Furthermore, it is suggested stores prepare to ramp up internet shopping and self-checkout to facilitate social distancing and lessening the threat of contracting the PI (Food Marketing Institute 2006). Ensuring employees in these industries remain safe during a pandemic is paramount to their ability in remaining viable in order to meet the needs of the public. Consequently, business continuity planning will assist all industries in mitigating the effects of PI and ensure individual communities' survival. A hospital cannot survive alone and needs the assistance of outside organizations and businesses to provide services to the facility in the form of electricity, water, medical gases, food, and other supplies.

Notwithstanding the preparation of government and private corporation mitigation for PI, it is vitally important for individuals to prepare for an upcoming pandemic. Everyones' best intentions will not completely prepare individual communities or this country for a pandemic, however, an individual's preparation coupled with the public and private entities will reduce the overall disruption that will occur. Private citizens should not rely on the government for support as it might not come. The widespread disaster will quickly overwhelm any relief effort and communities and their inhabitants will be left to themselves to overcome the pandemic. Emergency preparedness for families is not a new concept and should be revisited especially with increasing occurrences of natural disasters worldwide. A family that is prepared for disasters or even a pandemic will have much less to fear than those who did not prepare, which may prove to be the difference between life and death.

Individual emergency preparedness includes food and water supplies, medications, first aid supplies, and various other items to meet minimal requirements for survival. Many websites exist selling these types of supplies and provides ideas and creative means to maintain some level of comfort in a home during emergencies. A quick internet search will provide most individuals what they need to prepare themselves for emergencies, most of which is available at the local grocery or general merchandise store. The big concern is asking the question of what is needed or should be stored for such an emergency. A good guide for individuals to study is entitled *Pandemic Flu – Take The Lead Working Together to Prepare Now* and is published by the U.S. Department of Health and Human Services, which can be downloaded for free at www.takethelead.pandemicflu.gov. This document provides several checklists for families to review to assist in their preparation for future disasters and pandemics.

Additionally, individuals can follow several guidelines to minimize the chance of infection from a pandemic flu or any other type of illness. Limiting contact between persons in a technique called _social distancing' is one measure that could slow the spread of the disease. Furthermore, practicing good hygiene measures such as hand washing frequently, covering mouth and nose when coughing or sneezing, and the utilization of hand sanitizers will go a long way to diminish contact with a virus. Another, yet more invasive measure is to wear a facemask if you are ill that will assist in catching droplets of fluid that may contain the virus, but will do little to nothing if the virus is airborne. If airborne, a respirator can be worn to reduce the chance of being exposed to the flu or other virus (US Department of Health and Human Services n.d.). These universal precautions have been in use in the healthcare field for years and if performed properly will slow the transmission of the flu virus. Ultimately, individual preparedness and mitigation efforts will provide the greatest protection against a pandemic, which will assist in minimizing demand on the healthcare system. Hospitals actively instructing the public about individual precautions can minimize transmission and slow the spread of the virus.

Hosptial Viability

Arguably, the most difficult pandemic mitigation efforts will take place in hospitals. For a hospital to remain viable and ready to treat patients it will have to make preparations for increasing surge capacity, expediently credentialing new or volunteer providers, workforce management, maintaining essential services, logistics replenishment, security, and media communications. It is vitally important healthcare facilities prepare not only an ―all hazards" emergency operations plan (EOP), but also have a specific pandemic influenza (PI) plan. The usual EOP is meant for a short duration event not lasting much more than 96 hours, however, PI will last months before a vaccine is ready for mass prophylaxis. Therefore, if hospitals do not make preparations for longer duration events such as a pandemic, it will be almost impossible to provide safe and effective care to those who need it.

During a pandemic, it is expected that hospitals will surge the number of beds it can staff to care for the increased number who are ill. Surge capacity is defined as, ―a healthcare system's ability to rapidly expand beyond normal services to meet the increased demand for appropriate space, qualified personnel, medical care, and public health in the event of bioterrorism, disaster, or other large-scale, public health emergencies" (Dayton et al. 2008, 113). Many emergency responses will require

32

healthcare facilities to initiate their surge plans, but a pandemic is much different. One third of the world's population could become ill, including hospital workers.

> Current planning scenarios from the US Department of Health and Human Services anticipate that a flu pandemic would involve a minimum of 839,000 additional hospitalizations and an increase of at least 25% in demand for ICU beds and ventilators. Guidance suggests planning for such a surge in hospital demand by examining staffing issues, bed capacity, and the stockpiling of eight weeks of consumable supplies. (Avery et al. 2008, 2)

Surging in this environment with one third or more of a hospital's staff at home or in the hospital themselves will require facilities to think outside the box when developing a viable plan to surge during a pandemic. Possible answers include a fast credentialling process for non-hospital healthcare providers in outpatient settings to temporarily assist during the heightened demand peaks coiciding with the flu waves. Additionally, nursing schools or medical schools in the area might be willing to set up some type of supervised assistance to alleviate some of the staffing shortages. Unfortunately, these suggestions will be ripe with criticism due to legal aspects, but should be considered in the event of a pandemic (Avery et al. 2008).

When considering these and other non-traditional means of staffing, it is important to review an institution's human resource policies ensuring the facility maintain state and federal employment laws such as the Family and Medical Leave Act, the Americans with Disabilities Act and honor Health Insurance Portability and Accountability Act guidelines. Additionally, other legal concerns could be eliminated if the healthcare professionals register with the Emergency System for Advanced Registration of Volunteer Health Professionals (ESAR-VHP). This program is a registry for current healthcare volunteers and their credentialing information (Ransom, Goodman and Moulton 2008). Initiating requirements such as these for volunteers is a relatively simple task if done prior to the outbreak of a pandemic. However, not all problems with surge plans will be worked out prior to a pandemic, but a failure to plan is a plan to fail.

Another coinciding issue in workforce management is whether the healthcare staff will show up to work during a pandemic. Many believe the increased risk to the staff and their families during a pandemic will prevent them from coming to work. In Germany, a university hospital survey found that 28 percent of respondants felt it would be professionally acceptable for healthcare professionals to abandon their workplace during a pandemic to protect themselves and their families (Ehrenstein, Hanses and Salzberger 2006). Similarly, 89.7 percent of primary care providers surveyed in Singapore were worried they were at an increased risk for becoming ill with avian influenza; however, only 11.8 percent would consider stopping work (Wong et al. 2008). Furthermore, a study of mixed healthcare professionals in the U.S. revealed that up to 50 percent of healthcare workers would be unwilling to work during a pandemic outbreak, however, clinical staff would be more likely to attend than others (Draper et al. 2008). Moreover, 40 percent of healthcare workers polled in Maryland, would not attend work during a pandemic, but 86.8 percent of the physicians polled said they would attend (Siegel 2006). These surveys reveal a very real fear by healthcare workers for their own and families safety if they attend work during a pandemic outbreak.

Subsequently, it remains a management problem how to alleviate at least some of the fear to persuade not only the clinicians, but also the non-clinical workers to be present at work in such conditions. The hospital needs to assure the staff that provisions have been made for their families and the workers must feel like they are being protected as much as possible from the medical threat. Healthcare workers participating in a bioterrorism exercise responded to the question about what they could do differently during the exercise and they stated, ―Pre-planning for families of healthcare workers was thought to be crucial. Identifying secure locations for families to stay, potentially near the hospital, prioritizing family members for vaccine or prophylaxis, and arranging for childcare facilities were seen as high priorities‖ (Henning et al. 2004,149). The bottom line is if you plan to assist with the family members and try to protect them, the healthcare workers will be more likely to attend work.

Additionally, the staff needs to feel safe at work, while they are performing their duties. Healthcare facilities need to stockpile enough antiviral medication for several weeks of prophylaxis, at the very minimum, for the clinical staff and their families. This will allow time for the SNS of antiviral medications to be distributed for further assistance. Furthermore, when a vaccination for the virus is available, the hospital must plan to vaccinate the clinical staff, healthcare workers, and family members as soon as possible. It will be necessary to prioritize vaccination if enough doses are not available. Providing a prophylaxis dose of antiviral medication or vaccination will assist in alleviating fears of taking an illness home to the family (Nevada Hospital Association n.d.). Another safety measure that can alleviate fear is the provision of adequate personal protective equipment (PPE) for the staff to utilize. It will be necessary for the hospital to stockpile a significant supply of PPE, because as soon as a pandemic occurs the suppliers‘ warehouses will empty and it will be uncertain how fast more supplies will be available to purchase.

In addition, merely providing the supplies will not be enough to make the staff feel safe as indicated by nurses‘ beliefs during a public health emergency. Nurses fear abandonment due to past experiences with Hurricane Katrina and other recent disasters worldwide. ―Nurses believed that clinical settings would be chaotic, without a clear chain of command, and with some colleagues refusing to work. Limited access to PPE, risk of infection, unmanageable numbers of patients, and possibly being assaulted for their PPE resulted in the sense that they would be in unsafe clinical environments" (O'Boyle, Robertson and Secor-Turner 2006, 351). Therefore, hospitals will need to focus on security to ultimately protect their staff, equipment, and supplies, from violent acts. It is naive to believe that outside security forces will rush to every hospital to protect them during a pandemic. Law enforcement will be overwhelmed with a myriad of issues as well as, absenteeism, which will require prior planning on the hospitals' part to ensure adequate security is available during a public health emergency (Gonzalez 2002). It is possible during a PI outbreak that hospital security will be the key to ensuring a healthcare facility remains viable throughout the event. Thus, with the presence of adequate hospital security, staff members' fears will diminish.

There are two types of security available to hospitals, passive and active. Passive security involves leveraging technology to assist in limiting access within a hospital. Examples of passive security include proximity badges that unlock doors when a badge is swiped or comes within a certain distance from the sensor, key pads, closed circuit television, which records activity of individuals moving throughout the hospital, and biometrics, which requires storing fingerprint data or retinal scans to allow access to secured areas. Active security requires the employment of security guards to actively patrol grounds, check identification, and guard access points within a hospital. The deciding factor on which type or combination of options to choose when employing security is the cost. Passive security usually requires a significant initial purchase cost, but is relatively inexpensive to maintain. Active security requires more money over time due to the long-term salaries required to employ guards. A combination of the two security types is usually the best alternative when determining how to conduct security at a hospital. In addition, security measures need to be scalable to meet the threat facing the facility and balanced by the funds available. Thus, the hospital will still have weak points, but the administration will have to determine where they will accept risk and to what level. If the healthcare facility is in a rural farming community with a low crime rate, there is generally a modest need for active security. However, if it is a large metropolitan hospital located in a area associated with a high crime rate, security will require multiple solutions including active and passive measures (Blackwell 2006).

Active and passive security measures that are adequate during normal operations will require additional focus in emergency management situations. Unfortunately, many hospitals have not made any changes to their security protocol in their emergency operations plans. Security planning for emergencies begins when an organization performs a threat assessment or Hazard Vulnerability Analysis (HVA), which determines the most likely threats facing the facility and the estimated risk associated with the hazard. Hospitals are required to perform an HVA annually if they are accredited by the Joint Commission, which instituted this requirement in 2001 (Steinhauer and Bauer 2002). Understanding the threats a hospital faces in all types of disasters including manmade and natural is just the first step to ensuring the viability of the facility. Secondly, a security assessment should be conducted to determine a hospital's weaknesses and strong points. A free security assessment can be downloaded at http://www.iroquois.org/cmt/cf/documents/Hospital%20Security%20and%20Force%20P rotection.pdf and is located in Appendix B of the document. Consequently, understanding strengths and weakness of a facility's security and the threats it will likely face is the basis for creating a hospital security plan. The plan should focus on mitigating the threats from the HVA and employ security measures to reduce weak points in the hospital. Furthermore, upon completion of a security plan, it must be tested. Ensure security is involved in every disaster drill and perform spot checks to make certain any technical equipment is working properly (Blackwell 2006). Providing adequate security will keep patients and employees safe during normal operations, as well as emergencies.

Reducing the fears of staff and getting them to show up for work is a major hurdle, but not the only one to ensure the hospital remains viable during a pandemic outbreak. No doubt some services will have to be curtailed, especially elective procedures; however, the facility will need to maintain essential services for life saving and critical care capabilities. Dr. Michael Pietrzak (2004) describes these essential services as a hospital's _critical axis,' which includes:

1. The accident and emergency department (A&E)

2. Operating suites

3. Critical care and acute care beds

4. Imaging, laboratory and pharmacy capabilities (essential elements only)

5. Vital facility resources and supplies such as food service

6. Utilities such as water, medical gases, power, ventilation systems, etc.

7. Communications, infomatics

8. Command and control centers (Pietrzak 2004, 1)

Maintaining these services is essential to remaining viable during any emergency management event. It is beyond the scope of this study to explain in detail what needs to occur with each of these items mentioned in the critical axis, notwithstanding these should be essential elements of any hospital's EOP. The only difference during a pandemic is the critical axis may need outside augmentation for weeks or months, which will become a difficult, but essential task.

It is also necessary to plan for the replenishment of supplies during this long term public health disaster. Cost will always be a concern when dealing with logistical resupply, but when economic systems may be hanging by a thread due to absenteeism, it is likely hospitals will not be receiving regular compensation from insurance companies or private payers. Thus, the ability to purchase scarce medical supplies will be problematic. Many healthcare facilities are relying upon the state or federal government resources to bail them out in this situation, which may or may not be available in the time of need. It is essential that the facilities plan for redundancy of suppliers and a small stockpile until supplies are available for distribution (Avery et al. 2008). Consequently, even if all other preparations have been made, without an adequate logistics resupply, the hospital will not remain viable for operation.

One more way in which a hospital can maintain its operations is through the use of media communications. The opportunity for healthcare professionals to educate the general public in areas of hygeine, disenfection, and caring for a family member with influenza will prove invaluable in reducing the numbers of patients coming to the emergency department. Broadcast media maintain an important public service during an emergency and should be incorporated into every community plan for information dissemination (Cretikos et al. 2008). This vital role of the media could ultimately be the difference between public concern and civil unrest. In summary, to ensure a hospital remains viable during a pandemic outbreak, prior planning is necessary for surge capacity, provider credentialling, workforce management, security, critical axis elements, logistics, and media communications.

Domestic Security

Further insight is needed to determine the likelihood of outside response to hospitals during a pandemic outbreak. As previously stated, one should not depend on outside security forces to assist in providing security to healthcare institutions; however, past use of the military in civil disturbance incidents leads one to believe that some forces will be utilized to restore law and order when needed. Thus, it is necessary to examine the role of the military in domestic disorders. Additionally, as evident from Hurricane Katrina, contractors were utilized to defend private property from looters in New Orleans (Scahill 2005). Consequently, it is necessary to address the feasibility of private contractors securing a healthcare facility during a manmade or natural disaster.

The role of the military in domestic disorders has been under scrutiny for years, stemming from the Posse Comitatus Act, —Whoever, except in cases and under circumstances expressly authorized by the Constitution or Act of Congress, willfully uses any part of the Army or the Air Force as a posse comitatus or otherwise to execute the laws shall be fined under this title or imprisoned not more than two years, or both" (United States Code 1878). Originating from the election of 1876, which ended the period of reconstruction following the Civil War, the Act was meant as a protection for the federal troops to keep the U.S. marshals and sheriffs from conscripting the Army forces into posses for local law enforcement. Now, it would require the President to approve the use of federal military forces for local law enforcement activities. The Posse Comitatus Act does not prevent the President from using federal troops during riots or civil disorders, which can be overridden through the Insurrection Act in a crisis. In fact, federal troops have been used frequently over the years upholding and enforcing the law. Additionally, it does not prohibit the military from supporting local or federal law enforcement, except for investigating crimes or making the arrest of citizens (Brinkerhoff 2002). Much is misunderstood about the Posse Comitatus Act, which will likely force a change to the law in the near future.

The possibility of lawlessness during a pandemic influenza outbreak will likely invoke the president to utilize the military in this domestic disorder, thus the Posse Comitatus Act will require the President, or Act of Congress to approve their use. The possibility for disorder will occur when the healthcare facilities are overwhelmed and cannot take care of everyone seeking treatment, as people vie for medications or vaccines in limited supply, as persons compete for life sustaining necessities limited by broken logistics chains, and as people attempt to leave areas that have been quarantined for containment of the illness. Consequently, federal entities and military commands should be prepared to provide assistance in medical treatment, law enforcement, and border patrol functions (U.S. Department of Homeland Security 2006).

If doubt exists as to the probability of civil unrest occurring in the pandemic environment, then looking back in history to 1992 during the Los Angeles riots should dispel the uncertainty. The origins of the riot were from the arrest and beating of Rodney King, a black motorist, subsequent to a high-speed car chase in March of 1991. The white

41

and Hispanic officers involved were arrested and charged for their crimes against Mr. King. They were subsequently brought to trial and acquitted of their crimes. The news of their acquittal ignited the Los Angeles riots on 29 April 1992, for which 7,000 National Guardsmen were called into action to quell the rioting. Over the next several days, it was determined more assistance would be necessary, thus an additional 4,000 active duty military from the Marines and Army were called into action. The riot lasted five days and cost the lives of 54 persons and property damages exceeding $900 million dollars (Scheips 2005). Consequently, this example provides the illustration that it does not require a monumental act to spark civil unrest. The likelihood of increased fear coupled with survivalist instincts will be more than enough to be the catalyst for unrest. It is important that military leaders understand their roles and prepare for such assistance as needed.

Another possibility for law enforcement during a pandemic is the use of private contractors to secure public and private property. For years private contractors have assisted in Iraq and Afghanistan, so what will stop them from assisting during a pandemic or other disaster? In fact, they already have. In 2005, the Federal Government utilized Blackwater contractors to assist in providing security in New Orleans after Hurricane Katrina. Approximately 150 Blackwater security forces patrolled the streets in full tactical gear to include automatic weapons to secure neighborhoods and even confronted criminals (Scahill 2005). As the military continues to be stretched thin on two war fronts, contractors will remain an integral part of the security force. In some ways these contractors are not constrained by the same rules or laws, the military is and can be used for the benefit of the government. However, contractors or mercenaries, as some call them, can also bring vigilantism because the laws that govern them are not as strict.

Consequently, when contemplating the use of contractors it is very important to specify implicitly what their role is and the training needed to perform their mission. Additionally, the contractors must be a part of hospital emergency management exercises to ensure compliance with command and control, communications, and security roles during emergency management situations. Certainly, there exists a role for contractors performing security during disasters and other emergencies, but further guidance is necessary to determine the capabilities of this future asset. Summarily, domestic security performed by the military, contractors, and law enforcement agencies are faced with increasingly difficult questions of jurisdiction, enforcement capabilities, and tactics for dealing with domestic disorders in the new century. However, as the recent past has shown, each of these entities has a role in protecting the lives of citizens, establishing order, and protecting public and private property during disasters. Thus, it can be reasonably expected that the military and private security contractors will provide some assistance to hospitals during a pandemic.

In summary, pandemic influenza is a proven credible threat facing our country. In some cases, it seems like a doomsday scenario with no hope for overcoming its effects upon the world. However, if careful planning and preparation occur at all levels of government and in the CI/KR industries, much of the threat can be mitigated. Reviewing the current PI literature allows us to understand the complexities and importance of preparing ourselves for the future so our wonderful country and our public and private institutions can continue to prosper for generations to come. If we prepare as a healthcare industry now to meet the demands that will occur during a pandemic or other emergency, we will have no need to fear when the next disaster comes our way.

CHAPTER 3

RESEARCH METHODOLOGY

Research Design

This study will employ a comparative case study methodology utilizing four

prominent emergency management and public health events in the past century: 1918,

Spanish flu (H1N1); 2003, SARS outbreak; 2005, Hurricane Katrina, and the 2009,

Swine flu (H1N1) outbreak, which currently is not a pandemic. Thus, Hurricane Katrina,

and the other public health events will serve as the case studies while juxtaposing their

data to determine similarities and differences with regard to hospital viability measures

during the four phases of emergency management: mitigation, preparedness, response,

and recovery. Furthermore, the public health actions will be categorized as either

community based or hospital measures to distinguish patterns of relevancy. The case

study is meant to be exploratory in order to discover patterns of public health measures

that proved to be effective or ineffective in dealing with emergency management

situations.

The results from the case study will provide the basis of the hospital viability

checklist for PI that will assist healthcare facilities in mitigating threats during a PI

outbreak. Additional research may be required to complete the hospital viability checklist

in order to make it useful in the healthcare field today. Thus, this portion of the research

will be conducted utilizing current literature to fill any gaps the case study may leave out.

Moreover, the researcher will address the feasibility for the military or a private

contractor to conduct security at hospitals during the pandemic period. This multifaceted

45

approach to create the hospital viability checklist for PI will ensure a useful product that is relevant today in preparing for the next pandemic.

Primary Research Question

Understanding the emergency management process is the beginning to uncovering actions the healthcare industry should undertake during catastrophes. However, the "all hazards" approach is inadequate to respond to a moderate pandemic outbreak. Shortcomings of our fragile healthcare framework combined with the prolonged duration of a pandemic make it difficult to prepare for such a catastrophic disaster. Therefore, the purpose of this study is to determine, what should hospitals do to remain viable during a pandemic influenza outbreak?

Secondary Research Questions

To answer the primary research question, the following secondary questions should be addressed: Should either the military or private security be utilized to augment security at hospitals? What should hospitals do to encourage their employees to show up for work during an outbreak of Pandemic Influenza? What are the significant aspects of hospital security during a pandemic influenza outbreak? These questions are all significant, but the most important is the ability for a hospital to remain viable during a pandemic. Subsequently, it is difficult for a hospital to remain viable without addressing these secondary research questions. Thus, their importance exists as building blocks to determine how a hospital can continue keep its doors open during the largest and longest mass casualty event of most healthcare workers careers. The accumulation of the hospital viability measures coupled with its subsequent analysis will be the basis for answering

the study's questions and providing guidance to the healthcare industry today.

Data Collection & Analysis

This study will utilize a matrix designed to capture security measures undertaken

throughout the case studies (see Table 2).

Table 2.　Pandemic Case Study Viability Matrix

Viability Measure Implemented	1918 Pandemic (H1N1)	2003 SARS Outbreak	2005 Hurricane Katrina	2009 Swine Flu (H1N1)	Source(s)
Hospital Measures					*Measures are either things that did occur, current suggested measures, or measures to implement in the future from lessons learned
Mitigation = Long-term measure for reducing or elimiating risk					
Insert Measure Here					
Preparedness = A state of readiness					
Insert Measure Here					
Response = Reaction to an event aimed at containment or control					
Insert Measure Here					
Recovery = Return operations to their normal status					
Insert Measure Here					
Community Measures					
Insert Measure Here					
Mitigation = Long-term measure for reducing or elimiating risk					
Insert Measure Here					
Preparedness = A state of readiness					
Insert Measure Here					
Response = Reaction to an event aimed at containment or control					
Insert Measure Here					
Recovery = Return operations to their normal status					
Insert Measure Here					

Source:　Created by author.

The researcher will read histories, lessons learned, and other literature of each case study in order to find accounts of viability measures implemented during each disaster. These accounts will then be annotated on the matrix and marked with an –X" indicating the viability measure occurred during the specified case study. If an –X" is not listed beneath a specified case study, then it indicates the security measure was not indicated in the literature for that case. Any shortcomings from the data collection will be merged with current viability measures found in literature to complete the hospital viability checklist.

Significance

Most hospitals do not adequately address the need for security or other key measures during a Pandemic Influenza outbreak and are at risk of not remaining viable during an initial or subsequent wave of infection (Blackwell 2006). Many hospitals are leaving out numerous viability measures, which will lead to a lack of needed healthcare services during a PI occurrence. Therefore, a hospital viability checklist for pandemic influenza will be provided to assist in mitigating significant threats during an outbreak. Subsequently, if hospitals utilize the guidance provided in the checklist, their facilities will be better prepared in remaining viable throughout the pandemic. Thus, not only will a hospital be able to keep its doors open, but many lives will be saved.

Assumptions

Most if not all hospitals will become overwhelmed with patients during a pandemic influenza outbreak and will struggle to remain viable due to the poor planning of healthcare institutions to handle security or staffing in this time of need. Additionally, the Department of Defense has not adequately addressed the probable call for assistance to augment security at hospitals or pharmacies in the US.

Limitations

Due to the constrained time requirement for this study, no survey of healthcare workers to determine the likelihood of them attending work or factors that would encourage them to work during a pandemic will be conducted. Thus, current studies on this topic will be utilized. Another limitation is the ability to find the histories and AAR's that contain the viability measures, which could skew the results of the study. Additionally, the use of the 2009 H1N1 influenza epidemic is not fully underway and will limit the actions and responses noted in the comparative analysis; however, the current epidemic will bring to light modern practices for mitigating the effects of the next pandemic.

Delimitations

This study will not provide an all-inclusive answer about how to operate during emergency management operations, but will focus on how a hospital remains open and viable during a pandemic influenza outbreak. Additionally, legal concerns exist with medical volunteers and needs to be addressed, but will have to be answered by state and federal lawmakers in order to protect the volunteers and the healthcare facilities during emergency operations.

CHAPTER 4

ANALYSIS

The results of the study were more than expected partially because of the late decision to add the 2009 H1N1, swine flu epidemic, as a case study. Even though the epidemic had only recently emerged, the ability to synthesize public health measures enacted in Mexico and the United States was a great opportunity to evaluate the current preparedness levels and options for mitigating pandemic influenza (PI). The current WHO pandemic level is at five, meaning a pandemic is imminent. Hopefully, the results of this study will be made available prior to subsequent waves to allow time for healthcare facilities preparing themselves for possible mutations, which could increase the virulence causing more stress on the fragile healthcare framework (Barry 2005). Thus, answering this study's questions will offer pertinent guidance, which will assist hospitals in remaining viable during a pandemic. Subsequently, analyzing the results of the comparative case study and evaluating the results with the study's questions will demonstrate its usefulness to the emerging pandemic today.

Results

First, it is necessary to discuss the results of the comparative case study. The study identified viability measures contained within the case studies. A viability measure is a public health or hospital action designed to mitigate the effects of PI within the community at large or in healthcare facilities. After reviewing the case study literature, 117 viability measures were identified (see Appendix A). Out of the 117 viability measures, 96 or 82 percent were implemented or planned with respect to the 2009, H1N1

50

swine flu epidemic; 37 or 32 percent were implemented or suggested as lessons learned in regards to Hurricane Katrina; 35 or 30 percent were implemented or suggested as lessons learned with respect to the 2003, SARS epidemic; and 24 or 21 percent were implemented or suggested as lessons learned in response to the 1918, H1N1 Spanish flu pandemic. Additionally, only four viability measures out of 117 were found in common between all the case studies, while there were 11 measures, which were in common between three of the case studies. Furthermore, two case studies shared 41 viability measures and 61 measures were related to only one of the four cases (see figure 2).

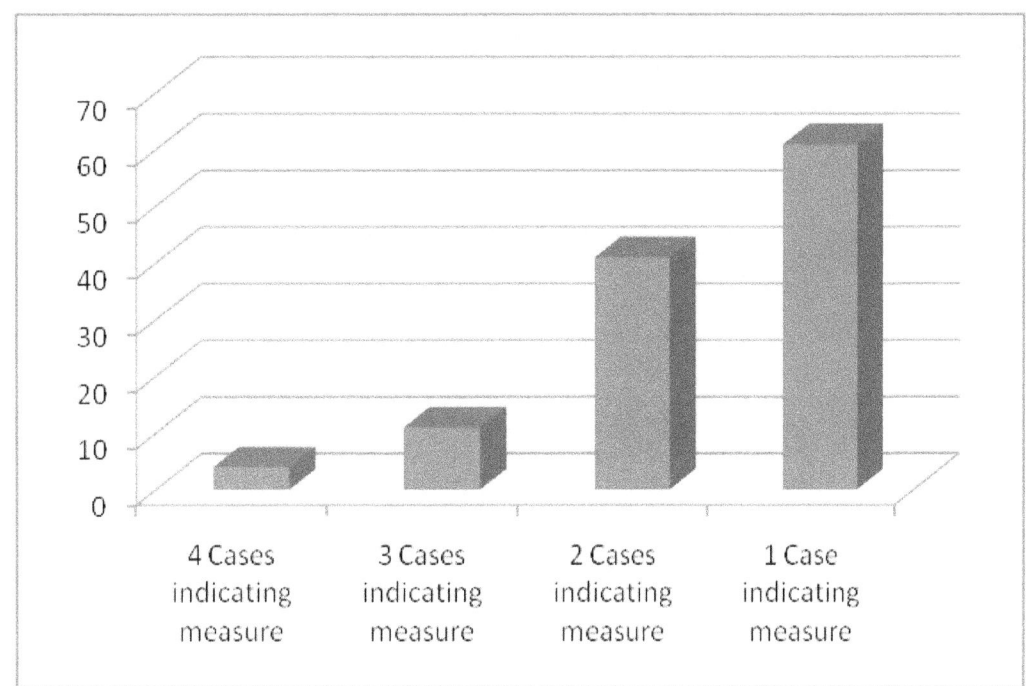

Figure 2.　Number of Cases per Measure

Source: Created by author.

Furthermore, the greatest correlation between the case studies was Hurricane Katrina and the 2009 Swine Flu with 26 percent of the measures indicated by each case. This is probably due to the many changes within emergency management in the past few years, which occurred after the 2003 SARS outbreak. The second highest correlation was between the 2009 Swine Flu and the 2003 SARS outbreak with 24 percent of the measures indicated by each case. The higher correlation between SARS and the 2009 Swine Flu was expected as they are similar public health emergencies; however, the SARS response lacked some of the latest techniques assisting in the mitigation and response of epidemics or pandemics. The rest of the cases indicated correlation of viability measures somewhere between 8 percent to 12 percent of the total measures found (see figure 3).

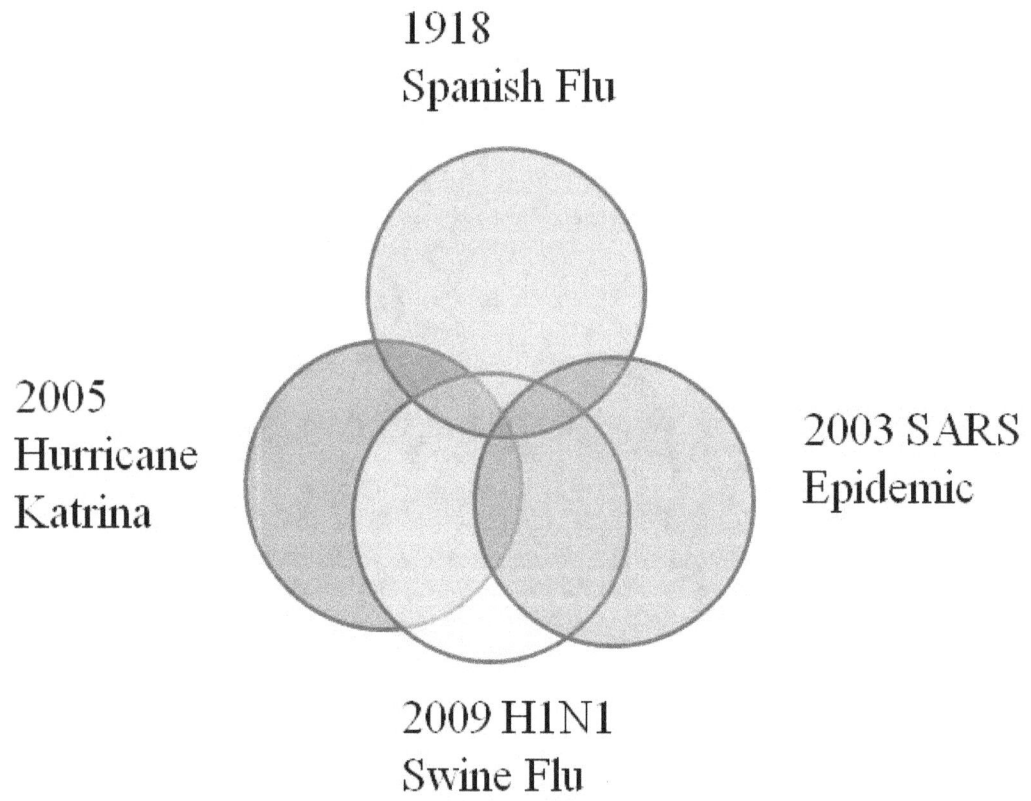

Figure 3.   Case Study Venn Diagram
Source: Created by author.

The importance of these figures lies within the commonality between the case studies. Thus, the individual viability measures that were found in common between all the case studies indicate several actions that should be present in all emergency management cases which were: the use of mass media to inform public of health and sanitation practices to reduce infection; government officials, experts, and media must be honest with public and work to discredit unwarranted fears; close schools; and cancel public events. Two of the four deal with information dissemination via the media from experts and government officials suggesting the power and value of engaging the media organizations in emergencies to distribute accurate and honest information. A caution does exist if the media is allowed to speculate about issues during the disaster, which will cause confusion and panic in the community. Therefore, it is paramount that key leaders and officials prepare to engage the media with accurate information and work to discredit fears that can cause panic (Barry 2005). The other two measures consisted of closing schools and cancelling public events, which are good things to do during a public health crisis, but happened to be coincidental during Hurricane Katrina due to the widespread damage that occurred.

Additionally, those measures occurring post disaster in at least three out of the four studies indicates relevance in employing that particular tactic during a pandemic today. Subsequently, these 11 measures combined with the other four previously mentioned are tested actions that worked in the past and will continue to be of benefit if implemented in the future. These 15 measures were consolidated into 10 measures, which include implementing the following:

1. Employ trained public affairs personnel to expertly engage the media and provide critical information to the public decreasing fear and increasing order

2. Coordinate with local media in order to provide the public with current and relevant information and education materials about a pandemic or other disaster

3. Develop an emergency operations plan (EOP) for organizations allowing preparedness to mitigate the effects of the disaster

4. Hospitals should develop a surge plan for mass casualty incidents, as well as, increased patient load due to an epidemic or pandemic

5. Organizations should exercise their EOP biannually in the form of disaster drills to test their preparedness and refine processes to better prepare for emergencies in the future

6. Provide mental health services to the first responders and hospital staff during and post disaster

7. Employ armed security forces at hospitals and key infrastructure to protect limited resources and promote civil order

8. Close schools, churches, cancel public events, etc. to limit the spread of a contagious virus (public health event)

9. Suggest voluntary isolation and quarantine of infected individuals and their families (public health event)

10. Wear N95 facemasks when in public to decrease the chance of spreading a pandemic flu (public health event)

The study produced many useful measures, but not all were implemented in every case study for several reasons. First, the 1918 Spanish flu pandemic exhibited many useful public health measures, which were instrumental in decreasing mortality in the large cities, but did not have the modern emergency management standards we enjoy today. Secondly, Hurricane Katrina provided insight about modern emergency management procedures, however, failed to discuss public health measures implemented during a pandemic. Even though many of the viability measures only appeared either by themselves or together in two cases, their importance should not be underestimated. In fact, the opposite occurred. Beginning with the 1918 pandemic, lessons learned have proliferated themselves with each new disaster from the process of evaluating what could be done differently during and after the event.

The result is suggestions and measures, which are constantly being refined. This is not to say all of our organizations are prepared for a pandemic, but many of these measures were implemented in isolation and are just now being compiled to bring together comprehensive preparedness plans for future events. The results from the case study in combination with current pandemic tools led to the development of The Hospital Pandemic Viability Checklist (see Appendix B). This checklist provides the healthcare community with a myriad of viability measures, which if implemented, will allow a hospital to remain open during the most austere environments including a moderate to severe pandemic. Not only is this important for a healthcare facilities financial bottom line, but also more importantly for the public to have a safe haven for refuge if needed. As a result, viability measures discovered in all of the cases hold value throughout emergency management events; however, it is the viability measures of the modern public health cases that will refine the mitigation efforts in the future response to PI.

How Do Hospitals Remain Viable During a Pandemic Influenza Outbreak?

Consequently, the results of the study provide the basis for answering the research questions posed. The primary research question is ―what should hospitals do to remain viable during a pandemic influenza outbreak?" The ability to answer this and the subsequent secondary questions lie partially in the case study matrix, which compared actions taken by hospitals and communities from the four historical emergency management events. The complete answer however, comes from the combination of information found within the case study matrix and the literature review, which provided the background on pandemic influenza. Thus, by combining these elements, several key measures became apparent in the ability for a hospital to remain viable during a pandemic: maintaining a hospital's critical axis, staffing, security, logistics, surge capacity, PAO campaign, and emergency plans. Four out of these seven measures came directly from the case study measures and were common across a minimum of three cases. The other three measures are from the literature review or case studies, but occurred in only one or two of the studies (See Table 3). Therefore, explaining how these measures will allow a hospital to remain viable during a pandemic will provide answers to the research questions.

Table 3.   Cross Reference of the Seven Pandemic Viability Measures

Viability Measure Implemented	1918 Pandemic (H1N1)	2003 SARS Outbreak	2005 Hurricane Katrina	2009 Swine Flu (H1N1)	Literature Review
1. Emergency Preparedness Planning		X	X	X	X
2. Employ armed security		X	X	X	X
3. Logistics stockpiles and redundant vendors for consumables			X	X	X
4. PAO media plan engaging media with accurate and honest information	X	X	X	X	X
5. Maintain the hospital's —Gitical Axis"					X
6. Hospital Staffing				X	X
7. Surge Capacity		X	X	X	X

Source: Created by author

A Hospital's Critical Axis

The first viability measure is to ensure the hospital maintains its essential services throughout the pandemic. Dr. Michael Pietrzak (2004) describes these essential services as a hospital's ‗critical axis,' which includes:

1. The accident and emergency department (A&E)

2. Operating suites

3. Critical care and acute care beds

4. Imaging, laboratory and pharmacy capabilities (essential elements only)

5. Vital facility resources and supplies such as food service

6. Utilities such as water, medical gases, power, ventilation systems, etc.

7. Communications, infomatics

8. Command and control centers (Pietrzak 2004, 1)

Without any of these services, a hospital's ability to care for its patients degrades very quickly, while others are so essential that a facility would have to close if it could not maintain them. For example, a facility's power plant, incuding water, medical gases, power, and ventilation is vital to the most basic hospital procedures. If any outside disruption occurs, the facility can only operate for about 96 hours without external support. In recent years the Joint Commission has increased requirements to be self sufficient for this minimal time in response to disasters like Hurricane Katrina (Nevada Hospital Association 2007). The Joint Commission's ―all hazards" approach certainly helps, but is not good enough for a severe pandemic. Consequently, ensuring the critical axis of a hospital remains operational is the first step in ensuring viability for the facility.

Hospital Staffing During Pandemic Influenza

The next measure is to maintain enough essential staff to provide services in the hospital. This does no good to have your critical axis operational if you do not have any staff to perform the roles required to sustain them, which brings up one of the secondary research questions, ―what should hospitals do to encourage their employees to show up for work during PI?" The study brought out several measures to encourage hospital staff to attend work, which were based on making the employee feel safe and taking care of their families. Things that would make the staffmember feel safe are ensuring there is enough personal protective equipment (PPE) to protect themselves, provide prophylaxis antivirals to boost their ability to fight off the virus, and provide security in the facility to protect them from patients who can become irrational in an environment of little resources. Additionally, providing for thier families is a good faith gesture by the hospital encouraging their staff to attend work in a dangerous environment. In addition, by providing the family with prophylaxis doses of antivirals the employee will be less worried about bringing the flu virus back into their home. For the same reason, it will be necessary to house some employees in a hotel away from their family to reassure them that their families are not at risk. Furthermore, single parents will need childcare enabling them to work as school closures are liklely during portions of the pandemic. Another issue that could keep staff from showing up is transportation. If public transportation is limited or shut down, it will be necessary to provide some sort of a shuttle service to provide rides to and from work. Planning for these measures and publicizing it with the hospital staff will reassure them that the facility has the employees best interest at mind, while they serve the general public during the pandemic.

Significant Aspects of Hospital Security During a PI Outbreak

Ensuring the safety of the employee is key for them to attend work. Subsequently, security plays the vital role in providing a safe and secure environment enabling the hospital to keep its doors open. One of the secondary research questions is ―what are the significant aspects of hospital security during a PI outbreak?" Current literature combined with this study provides eight measures in response to this question. This is not all-inclusive, but provides basic security measures allowing a hospital to maintain a safe and secure environment. The eight security measures to ensure viability are:

1. Limiting the entrances to one point of access where the patients can be funneled and then routed to the appropriate service or location

2. Limiting access to patients and their family members, unless a visitor has an authorized purpose such as a contractor providing services

3. Issue visitor badges or patient bands to differentiate access needs within the facility

4. Ensure numerous, adequate, and descriptive signage of current PI processes to provide guidance and direction for patients and visitors to follow

5. Employ armed security guards at the entrance of the facility to assist in guiding patients, providing face masks, issuing badges, and checking for contriband or weapons

6. Employ armed security guards at the pharmacy to protect the limited stocks of medications used during a PI outbreak

7. Employ armed security in the Emergency Department, especially if utilizing another entrance for influenza patients

8. During preparedness phase, ensure security guards participate in all hospital disaster drills

It is not necessary to discuss in detail the tenets of each measure, but to provide general guidance with respect to security during a pandemic. It is also important to note that the response must be scaleable, if the current situation does not warrant all of the suggested measures, then implement what is needed. However, constant monitoring of the situation is required as things can change very quickly.

First, access needs to be limited and can be accomplished through several methods. Security guards are the first hospital employees that the patients should see to reassure them of their safety and commitment to order within the facility. It is far easier to limit the entrances of a hospital to one, but however many are open, they must be manned to issue guidance and direction. Additionally, visitor badges assist staff members in limiting access to the critical axis or high security areas within the facility. It is easier to keep patients and visitors out of unauthorized areas if they are identified by an visitor badge. Consequently, as most facilities already practice, it is important for the staff to wear name badges identifying who they are. Secondly, security guards must be armed during a pandemic. As resources become scarce, individuals are more likely to do and say things that under normal social conditions would be considered deplorable and ultimately unlawful. For this reason, it is of great importance that security guards are trained in the detention of unlawful persons until law enforcement can arrive and make an arrest. A third point is that security does not always have to be active, meaning a security guard present, but can be passive, such as the use of security cameras. Passive security can be effective in the event there are not enough guards to perform all functions, but a fast response to incidences is ultimately required. These points of hospital security are only the most basic elements that should be implemented. Many more measures exist, which would benefit a hospital, not just during a pandemic. They can be found in the hospital pandemic viability checklist (see Appendix B).

The Utilization of Military and Contractor Security During a Pandemic

Another issue and secondary research question is should either the military or private security be utilized to augment security at hospitals during a pandemic? The simple answer is yes, based upon the incidences found in the case studies and DOD policy in the literature review. The case studies noted contracted security with automatic weapons standing at the front of hospitals in Mexico as a show of force during the initial panic of the 2009 H1N1 swine flu outbreak (Penhaul 2009). Additionally, in Louisiana during the aftermath of Hurricane Katrina private military security guards were utilized to secure buildings and deter looting within New Orleans (Scahill 2005). Privatized paramilitary security contractors may be an alternative to the National Guard or active duty forces if they are not available for service. Contracts should be made prior to a pandemic occurring to ensure availability of contractors when needed.

Furthermore, DOD forces have the mission to provide transportation and security during the distribution of the SNS stockpile. This has already occurred in the initial SNS distribution for the H1N1 flu in May of this year. Military forces also have the mission to provide security during a large-scale vaccination program entailing transportation, distribution, and security of the hospitals or clinics providing the mass vaccination. The final mission tasked to the military is to restore order in the case of civil instability (Department of Defense 2006). A moderate to severe pandemic will require the use of private contractors or military to secure medications, vaccinations, and provide much needed security during certain operations. The only question is on what scale with these forces be utilized. This will all depend on the need of the communities and the availability of forces required in the provision domestic security.

Logistics During a Pandemic

Just as security ensures peace and protection for the hospital, logistics provides the ability to treat patients. The best doctor in the world will have a difficult time saving lives if he does not have the appropriate materials on hand, thus the healthcare facility needs to ensure they stockpile frequently used supplies. As the study inicated in the comparative case study matrix, it is suggested hospitals stockpile a minimum of eight weeks of consumable supplies prior to the occurrence of a pandemic (Avery et al. 2008). This is contrary to the recent business practice, which minimizes supply inventories to cut costs called ‟just in time logistics". Some institutions will need to revamp their strategic plans enabling them to make the suggested logistical preparations. Funding sources are

62

available through DHS to prepare for pandemic influenza outbreaks and can be used to purchase certain supplies to stockpile. The stocks should be rotated to ensure these precious commodities do not expire and are available when they are needed. Additionally, healthcare facilities should secure multiple contracts with suppliers to ensure goods are available during a PI outbreak. Logistics are the lifeblood to the hospital, which without supplies will wither and die, or as in this case will no longer be viable for patient care.

Surge Capacity

Another key component the study found was that bed space, or surge capacity, was vital in the response to a pandemic. Every hospital should create or update a surge plan on an annual basis. Critics on both sides of the argument cannot be sure what will occur during a pandemic, but one thing is sure, if no plan exists, chaos will ensue. Certainly, surging capacity may free up beds and ventilators for use, but it will not guarantee there will be staff to treat the patients. Critics make the point that clinical staff will be ill and contracted hourly workers will be unavailable for hire during this immense demand period. Proponents suggest having volunteers register with state and National emergency management registries to create large pools of manpower that can be mobilized in affected areas. Additionally, legal issues abound with questions of training and credentialing of healthcare workers who will be rapidly called into action. There exist many options for increasing surge capacity and hospitals need to analyze options local to their community. None should be off the table, unless it would be illegal, immoral, or unethical. A severe pandemic will stretch the current healthcare infrastructure to the breaking point and hospital leadership needs to make every effort possible to ensure the doors do not close to patients seeking care.

Public Affairs

As hospitals attempt to surge, respond to the pandemic threat, or provide guidance to the community, they will require a public affairs campaign and an experienced staff member to manage it. Public affairs and the media have been involved in virtually every disaster of the last century. Certainly, not all disasters involved public health concerns, but the media played an important role disseminating information. The concern is that not all media messages assist in deminishing the threat or problems occurring. In fact, sometimes the media message incites panic and fear. For this reason, it is vitally important local leaders provide accurate, honest, and beneficial information to the media for dissemination to the public. The study recognized this as a key to remaining viable during a pandemic. Thus, it is not just the fact media puts out information, but of greater importance the information disseminated provides guidance about what the public can do to protect themselves and their families.

Emergency Operations Planning

The last viability measure encompasses all of the previous actions as they become encorporated into emergency plans. Consequently, planning is the most important measure because it provides a basic outline of how to function during emergencies. All of the case studies except for the 1918 Spanish flu utilized emergency management plans as a baseline for their response. These plans are called different things, recently the joint commission suggested the term emergency management plan be changed to emergency operations plan (EOP) (The Joint Commission 2008). An organization cannot necessarily manage an emergency, but they can operate in one and thus, the reason for the name change. The emergency operations plan will usually incorporate all planning for disasters and emergencies standing as an ―all hazards‖ plan, but pandemic influenza is so intensive that it requires its own plan. Today, hospitals utilize the hospital incident command system (HICS) as a command and control system that has specific job functions for hospital. This system is in synch with NIMS, which allows all the responders to speak the same language. The utilization of these planning systems in the development of a hospital‘s emergency operation plan creates synchronization within the community, establishes agreements between agencies, and provides a baseline of actions from which to function. If used properly, planning sets the stage for all other emergency management functions.

Emergency planning establishes a preparedness level within an organization that offers protections from disasters and enables the organization to remain viable during the catastrophe. Pandemic influenza planning differs slightly from basic emergency management planning due to the duration of the disaster. Thus, answering this study‘s question of how can a hospital remain viable during a pandemic influenza outbreak, does not introduce new technologies or concepts, but merges individual public health actions modeled after past emergency management cases and lessons learned to establish hospital viability measures. Therefore, to ensure a hospital will remain viable during a pandemic, the facility must maintain its critical axis, provide safety measures for the employee and their family, employ security to ensure safety of patients and staff, maintain stockpiles of consumable supplies and medications, retain surge capacity, prepare a public affairs campaign for PI, and continually improve and practice the EOP. Many other measures exist to enhance these hospital viability measures, however, these few act as a baseline from which to expand and should be considered the minimal approach to ensuring hospital viability. In contrast, a more comprehensive approach to maintaining hospital viability during a pandemic is contained within the hospital pandemic viability checklist. The checklist is the resulting product from the study and should be seen as the pinnacle of this research.

CHAPTER 5

CONCLUSIONS AND RECOMMENDATIONS

In the past 8 years since September 11, many improvements have been made to the national response capabilities; however, the ―all hazards‖ approach is still inadequate to respond to a moderate or severe pandemic outbreak. Shortcomings of our fragile healthcare framework coupled with the prolonged duration of a pandemic make it difficult to prepare for such a catastrophic disaster. Therefore, the purpose of this study was to investigate the factors ensuring hospital viability during a pandemic influenza outbreak. To accomplish this, the project employed a comparative case study for the purpose of finding common measures enabling a hospital and community to mitigate, prepare, respond, and recover from a disaster such as PI. The study discovered addressing seven common viability measures will assist in mitigating a moderate pandemic. The seven viability measures are:

1. Preparedness Planning

2. Employ armed security during a PI

3. Logistics stockpiles and redundant vendors for consumables

4. PAO media plan engaging media with accurate and honest information

5. Maintain the hospital's ―critical axis‖

6. Ensure the safety of the hospital's staff and their families

7. Create a hospital surge plan specific to a community

Moreover, a more comprehensive approach to preparing for a PI outbreak would be to utilize the hospital pandemic viability checklist (See Appendix B) as a guide to ensuring the healthcare facility is able to keep its doors open throughout the disaster. This checklist should not be viewed as an answer for solving every issue in regards to a pandemic, but is a good starting point to alleviate the heavy burden of researching how to mitigate, prepare, respond, and recover from such an emergency.

Furthermore, many hospitals lack the funding to prepare adequately for PI. This problem is increasing due to uncompensated care, poor insurance reimbursement, inflation, regulatory requirements, and workforce shortages. This vital healthcare resource will not be available during a pandemic, unless an organization is financially stable and willing to make the necessary preparations to mitigate a pandemic threat. Some funding is available, to assist hospitals in their preparation, but is not enough to fully prepare for such a disaster. Therefore, it is imperative a hospital begin preparations as soon as possible by slowly building up stocks of medications and consumable supplies to decrease an immediate financial burden.

Consequently, if the current Federal funding is insufficient for making preparations in case of a PI outbreak, then it is important for hospitals to seek assistance through state representatives in suggesting further legislation to increase funding in this area. Additional Federal legislation is needed for the funding of treatment in response to PI, which would alleviate fears of trying to recoup billions in uncompensated care. Similarly, legislators should consider issuing guidance in response to rationing of care, if the need exceeds the capability to provide adequate healthcare to the public. Hospital's ethics committees are struggling in the creation of treatment policies due to the current level of malpractice claims in the United States and need guidance or laws to protect the healthcare community in such catastrophic cases. Furthermore, the ability for hospitals to surge beyond normal capacity will be in part due to staffing and legal aspects to providing care offsite in non-healthcare settings such as churches or gyms. A comprehensive emergency response law should be enacted to protect the healthcare workers from liability in such disastrous conditions, which would reassure providers to show up to work and do the best job they can with the resources on hand.

For Further Study

Another issue that needs more research and attention is the utilization of paramilitary contractors providing hospital security a pandemic. Certainly, their use will prove advantageous, as it was during Hurricane Katrina in providing security in New Orleans, but federal legislation needs to set limits on their abilities to deter vigilante justice. With the proper guidelines, these private paramilitary organizations could alleviate the pressure on the overextended National Guard and full-time military units during such emergencies. Securing our Nation's critical infrastructure and key resources during a pandemic or any emergency is the key to our ability as a nation to recover from its effects. Thus, securing our nation's healthcare framework is the key to recovering from a moderate to severe pandemic. Time will tell if the current H1N1 strain will mutate to a more virulent form increasing the severity of the pandemic. Therefore, it is critical to prepare now in an effort to mitigate the threats of PI and other emergencies in preserving our healthcare capabilities of the future.

In addition, further research needs to occur as to whether hospital workers would be willing to attend work during a moderate or severe pandemic. Initially, it was the intention of this study to perform a survey of hospital employees to answer questions that current surveys leave out, such as, what actions performed by the healthcare facility

69

would make the employee feel safer and more likely to attend work? Most current studies just ask general questions as to perceived intentions of attendance during a pandemic. They leave out what could change perceptions to attend or deter them from showing up to work. This subject is even more important to address than the other measures as it is the only one the hospital and administration does not make the final decision, but the employee who determines their own action. Ensuring the healthcare staff members feel safe at work during a pandemic is no small task and effort should be made prior to the emergency or only the truly dedicated will show up.

In Summary, the very essence of what hospitals stand for is in jeopardy if the current H1N1 threat becomes more virulent on its pandemic journey. There is no doubt the H1N1, Swine Flu will become a pandemic, the question is how lethal will it become. The healthcare industry should not maintain a false sense of security because the effects of the Swine Flu are not severe, but should prepare as if it will become so. This virus is one mutation away from becoming more lethal or possible reassortment with the H5N1 Avian Flu allowing it to freely move from person to person. Either way, it is important to do all that we can now, to prepare for the future. Following the guidance provided in this study and improving on a facility's viability measures will strengthen it against this current and future threat of pandemic influenza.

GLOSSARY

Avian Flu: Avian or bird flu is caused by influenza viruses that occur naturally among wild birds. The H5N1 variant is deadly to domestic fowl and is transmissible from birds to humans. There is no human immunity and no vaccine is available (U.S. Department of Homeland Security 2006, 11).

Emergency Management (management focus): The science of managing complex systems and multidisciplinary personnel to address emergencies and disasters, across all hazards and through the phases of mitigation, preparedness, response, and recovery (The Institute for Crisis, Disaster, and Risk Management (ICDRM) at the George Washington University (GWU); for the Veterans Health Administration (VHA)/US 2006, 1-19).

Epidemic: A pronounced clustering of cases of disease within a short period of time; more generally, a disease whose frequency of occurrence is in excess of the expected frequency in a population during a given time interval (U.S. Department of Homeland Security 2006, 206).

Hospital Incident Command System (HICS): HICS is a methodology for using ICS in a hospital/healthcare environment. HICS is an incident management system based on the Incident Command System (ICS), that assists hospitals in improving their emergency management planning, response, and recovery capabilities for unplanned and planned events. HICS is consistent with ICS and the National Incident Management System (NIMS) principles. HICS will strengthen hospital disaster preparedness activities in conjunction with community response agencies and allow hospitals to understand and assist in implementing the 17 Elements of the hospital-based NIMS guidelines. HICS products include a Guidebook and planning and training tools (Emergency Medical Services Authority 2006).

Incident Command System (ICS): ICS is a standardized on-scene incident management concept designed specifically to allow responders to adopt an integrated organizational structure equal to the complexity and demands of any single incident or multiple incidents without being hindered by jurisdictional boundaries (The National Response Team 2000, 9).

National Incident Management System (NIMS): The National Incident Management System provides a systematic, proactive approach to guide departments and agencies at all levels of government, nongovernmental organizations, and the private sector to work seamlessly to prevent, protect against, respond to, recover from, and mitigate the effects of incidents, regardless of cause, size, location, or complexity, in order to reduce the loss of life and property and harm to the environment (US Department of Homeland Security 2008, 1).

Pandemic Influenza: A flu (influenza) pandemic is an outbreak of a new flu virus that spreads around the world. The virus will spread easily from person to person, mostly through coughing and sneezing. Because the virus is new to people, everyone will be at risk of getting it (US Department of Health and Human Services n.d., 3).

Personal protective equipment (PPE): PPE refers to the respiratory equipment, garments, and barrier materials used to protect rescuers and medical personnel from exposure to biological, chemical, and radioactive hazards (Horton et al. 2008, 105).

Physical Security: Physical security can be defined as that part of security concerned with physical measures designed to safeguard personnel, to prevent unauthorized access to equipment, material, installations and documents. It is also to safeguard against espionage, sabotage, damage and theft (SMT Security 2008).

Seasonal Flu: Seasonal or common flu is a respiratory illness that can be transmitted person to person. Most people have some immunity, and a vaccine is available (U.S. Department of Homeland Security 2006, 11).

Surge Capacity: A healthcare system's ability to rapidly expand beyond normal services to meet the increased demand for appropriate space, qualified personnel, medical care, and public health in the event of bioterrorism, disaster, or other large-scale, public health emergencies (Dayton et al. 2008, 113).

Viability Measure: A viability measure is a public health or hospital action designed to mitigate the effects of pandemic influenza within the community at large or in healthcare facilities.

APPENDIX A

CASE STUDY

APPENDIX B

HOSPITAL VIABILITY CHECKLIST FOR PANDEMIC INFLUENZA

Hospital Viability Measure:	Compliance IP – In Progress N/A – Not Applicable	Date Initiated	Compliance or Reassessment Date	Actions Required
Mitigation Phase				
1. Stockpile enough antiviral medication and antibiotics for staff and their families	☐ Yes ☐ No ☐ IP ☐ N/A			
2. Conduct Hazard Vulnerability Analysis (HVA)	☐ Yes ☐ No ☐ IP ☐ N/A			
3. Implement the use of Electronic Health Records (EHR)	☐ Yes ☐ No ☐ IP ☐ N/A			
4. Stockpile a minimum of 2 weeks antiviral medication, antibiotics, and PPE to enable distribution of SNS	☐ Yes ☐ No ☐ IP ☐ N/A			
5. Stockpile essential items such as PPE and respiratory items. Supplies may be difficult to obtain (maintain 2wk supply)	☐ Yes ☐ No ☐ IP ☐ N/A			
6. Maintain redundant communication systems with local and regional responders	☐ Yes ☐ No ☐ IP ☐ N/A			
7. Propose State and Federal legislation to provide for the funding of healthcare institutions during public health emergencies	☐ Yes ☐ No ☐ IP ☐ N/A			

Hospital Viability Measure:	Compliance IP – In Progress N/A – Not Applicable	Date Initiated	Compliance or Reassessment Date	Actions Required
8. Assist and lead if necessary in the development of the community response plan for pandemic influenza engaging community leaders and businesses in a collaborative effort	☐ Yes ☐ No ☐ IP ☐ N/A			
9. In accordance with local public health department, develop an emergency quarantine and isolation plan with local facilities that could be used to house people in the event of a large-scale quarantine	☐ Yes ☐ No ☐ IP ☐ N/A			
10. In coordination with local public health, maintain Global Outbreak Alert and Response Network (GOARN) and Global Public Health Intelligence Network (GPHIN) to network with State and National surveillance	☐ Yes ☐ No ☐ IP ☐ N/A			
11. Assist local public health department in the dissemination of influenza prevention measures	☐ Yes ☐ No ☐ IP ☐ N/A			
12. Hospital is up to date with general security measures for your local area (Urban hospitals should employ more measures than rural hospitals)	☐ Yes ☐ No ☐ IP ☐ N/A			
a. All doors and entrances monitored by CCTV	☐ Yes ☐ No ☐ IP ☐ N/A			

Hospital Viability Measure:	Compliance IP – In Progress N/A – Not Applicable	Date Initiated	Compliance or Reassessment Date	Actions Required
b. There is adequate security in the pharmacy to alleviate unauthorized access (Card access or keypad, locks, and CCTV)	☐ Yes ☐ No ☐ IP ☐ N/A			
c. All high-risk areas are monitored by CCTV	☐ Yes ☐ No ☐ IP ☐ N/A			
d. Lab restricts access by a locking mechanism (Lock, keypad, card access, etc).	☐ Yes ☐ No ☐ IP ☐ N/A			
e. Facility employees / volunteers use color photo ID badges: Name on the badge is large enough to read easily and depicts department, title, credentials (MD, RN, etc) and expiration date	☐ Yes ☐ No ☐ IP ☐ N/A			
f. Visitors show ID and sign-in and out and receive a visitor or out-patient badge. They are informed that the badge must be visible at all times.	☐ Yes ☐ No ☐ IP ☐ N/A			
g. Medical records are secured and have limited access in accordance to HIPAA standards (use of locks, keypad, or card access technologies).	☐ Yes ☐ No ☐ IP ☐ N/A			
h. Hospital is in compliance with HAZMAT / OSHA standards for sensitive items storage; thus all biohazard materials placed in locked freezers, incubators, and cabinets when not in use	☐ Yes ☐ No ☐ IP ☐ N/A			

Hospital Viability Measure:	Compliance IP – In Progress N/A – Not Applicable	Date Initiated	Compliance or Reassessment Date	Actions Required
i. Video surveillance of parking areas (CCTV) monitored 24 hours a day and roving guards provide physical exterior security on a regular basis	☐ Yes ☐ No ☐ IP ☐ N/A			
j. Air intake and HVAC systems are located at least 15ft off the ground and covered by metal grates. If system is on the roof, ensure exterior ladders are secured by a locking cage	☐ Yes ☐ No ☐ IP ☐ N/A			
k. Hospital's power plant including generator, telephone, and water supply is physically secured by fencing, locks and video surveillance (CCTV) monitored 24 hours a day	☐ Yes ☐ No ☐ IP ☐ N/A			
l. Guards conduct daily checks of security measures such as fencing, locks, CCTV, etc. to ensure proper working order	☐ Yes ☐ No ☐ IP ☐ N/A			
m. Agreement / MOU with local law enforcement to augment security for crowd control during emergency operations	☐ Yes ☐ No ☐ IP ☐ N/A			
n. Security Manager or consultant conducts annual security assessment and security committee reviews issues at least quarterly to ensure identification and solution of security shortcomings	☐ Yes ☐ No ☐ IP ☐ N/A			

Hospital Viability Measure:	Compliance IP – In Progress N/A – Not Applicable	Date Initiated	Compliance or Reassessment Date	Actions Required
o. Maintain Joint Commission standards for hospital security	☐ Yes ☐ No ☐ IP ☐ N/A			
p. Security communications are adequate and able to maintain contact with other guards and facilities Emergency Operation Center (EOC)	☐ Yes ☐ No ☐ IP ☐ N/A			
13. ED security policy to include calling security when a patient arrives with a GSW or penetrating wound	☐ Yes ☐ No ☐ IP ☐ N/A			
a. Metal detector in place at entrance to assist in confiscation of weapons (consider for larger metropolitan areas or history of gang activity)	☐ Yes ☐ No ☐ IP ☐ N/A			
b. Policies in place and staff trained to respond to weapons brought in by patients, visitors, staff, and law enforcement	☐ Yes ☐ No ☐ IP ☐ N/A			
c. A ―clearing barrel" used to safely clear confiscated weapons	☐ Yes ☐ No ☐ IP ☐ N/A			
d. Ambulance entrance door secured with keypad, card access, or constant security and local emergency responders given access	☐ Yes ☐ No ☐ IP ☐ N/A			
e. Minimum standoff distance for private vehicles of 25 meters (See UFC 4-010-01).	☐ Yes ☐ No ☐ IP ☐ N/A			

Hospital Viability Measure:	Compliance IP – In Progress N/A – Not Applicable	Date Initiated	Compliance or Reassessment Date	Actions Required
f. ED bay doors treated with anti-shard glass film / blast resistant capabilities	☐ Yes ☐ No ☐ IP ☐ N/A			
g. ED has separate restrooms and cafeteria / vending machines to reduce unauthorized persons in restricted areas	☐ Yes ☐ No ☐ IP ☐ N/A			
h. All entrances to ED monitored by CCTV or other passive or active monitoring system	☐ Yes ☐ No ☐ IP ☐ N/A			
Preparedness Phase				
1. Key leaders trained to utilize Hospital Incident Command System (HICS) and familiar with National Incident Management System (NIMS) processes during a disaster	☐ Yes ☐ No ☐ IP ☐ N/A			
2. Plan to provide childcare for staff members as schools may be out with no alternative	☐ Yes ☐ No ☐ IP ☐ N/A			
3. Plan to provide some basic necessities for employees such as food and water if quarantined away from their families	☐ Yes ☐ No ☐ IP ☐ N/A			
4. Plan to provide lodging for key staff to ensure they do not transmit virus to their families	☐ Yes ☐ No ☐ IP ☐ N/A			
5. Create / update Emergency Management Plan (EMP)	☐ Yes ☐ No ☐ IP ☐ N/A			

Hospital Viability Measure:	Compliance IP – In Progress N/A – Not Applicable	Date Initiated	Compliance or Reassessment Date	Actions Required
a. Create / update Hospital Pandemic Influenza (PI) Plan by pandemic phase classified by the World Health Organization (WHO)	☐ Yes ☐ No ☐ IP ☐ N/A			
b. Create / update Hospital Security Plan	☐ Yes ☐ No ☐ IP ☐ N/A			
c. Create / update Hospital Surge Capacity Plan	☐ Yes ☐ No ☐ IP ☐ N/A			
d. Create / update Morgue Surge Plan indicating a place in the hospital that can be used as a temporary surge site	☐ Yes ☐ No ☐ IP ☐ N/A			
e. Create ethical triage plan based upon probability of survival in limited resource environment (Phone triage, patient tracking, medical evacuation, triage location, etc)	☐ Yes ☐ No ☐ IP ☐ N/A			
f. Create / update mental health plan that deals with treating mentally ill during a pandemic	☐ Yes ☐ No ☐ IP ☐ N/A			
g. Create / update hospital vaccine distribution plan (Providers, nurses, etc.; plan for vaccine to be available 6-9 months after outbreak)	☐ Yes ☐ No ☐ IP ☐ N/A			
h. Create / update Business Continuity Plan see sample at www.docstoc.com	☐ Yes ☐ No ☐ IP ☐ N/A			
i. Designate a person as the pandemic influenza preparedness coordinator	☐ Yes ☐ No ☐ IP ☐ N/A			

Hospital Viability Measure:	Compliance IP – In Progress N/A – Not Applicable	Date Initiated	Compliance or Reassessment Date	Actions Required
j. Create an internal multidisciplinary team to assist the pandemic influenza coordinator in the planning and execution of the PI Plan	☐ Yes ☐ No ☐ IP ☐ N/A			
k. Members of the team should include a representative from: administration, legal, infection control, emergency manager, risk management, nursing, medical staff, ICU, ED, lab, pharmacy, radiology, mental health, respiratory therapy, environmental services, reception, public relations, security, logistics, staff development, occupational health, information technology, human resources, and a representative from the local public health department	☐ Yes ☐ No ☐ IP ☐ N/A			
l. Create / update a plan for rapid training of non-facility staff brought in to provide patient care when the hospital reaches surge capacity	☐ Yes ☐ No ☐ IP ☐ N/A			
m. Create / update facility access plan determining limiting of entrances, visitor access, lockdown procedures, visitor badges, staff badges, etc.	☐ Yes ☐ No ☐ IP ☐ N/A			

Hospital Viability Measure:	Compliance IP – In Progress N/A – Not Applicable	Date Initiated	Compliance or Reassessment Date	Actions Required
n. Obtain copies of relevant sections of the HHS Pandemic Influenza (PI) Plan and policy documents and review for incorporation into the facilities PI plan (see www.hhs.gov/pandemicflu/plan and www.pandemicflu.gov)	☐ Yes ☐ No ☐ IP ☐ N/A			
o. Obtain copies of other relevant PI plans and review (State, regional, local, tribal, etc.)	☐ Yes ☐ No ☐ IP ☐ N/A			
p. Develop PI plan actions based upon the World Health Organization (WHO)'s pandemic phases explained at www.who.int	☐ Yes ☐ No ☐ IP ☐ N/A			
q. Create / update communications plan addressing information for the media, public, healthcare workers, local government, and high risk groups	☐ Yes ☐ No ☐ IP ☐ N/A			
r. Develop Business Continuity Plan (Recovery)	☐ Yes ☐ No ☐ IP ☐ N/A			
6. Conduct Disaster Drills (Bi-Annually, Free tool at www.ahrq.gov for evaluation of drills)	☐ Yes ☐ No ☐ IP ☐ N/A			
a. Ensure security guards participate in disaster drills	☐ Yes ☐ No ☐ IP ☐ N/A			
b. Request Federal funding for disaster drills at www.dhs.gov	☐ Yes ☐ No ☐ IP ☐ N/A			

Hospital Viability Measure:	Compliance IP – In Progress N/A – Not Applicable	Date Initiated	Compliance or Reassessment Date	Actions Required
7. Ensure availability of mental health and religious services to hospital employees during the pandemic	☐ Yes ☐ No ☐ IP ☐ N/A			
8. Ensure facility has the capability to receive Emergency Alert System (EAS) messages	☐ Yes ☐ No ☐ IP ☐ N/A			
9. Maintain paper base capabilities for patient records and patient tracking in case of computer or power failure	☐ Yes ☐ No ☐ IP ☐ N/A			
10. Maintain emergency contact information for local, State, and Federal agencies and ensure the hospital EOC has them posted	☐ Yes ☐ No ☐ IP ☐ N/A			
11. Maintain key and essential personnel contact list and their back-ups with phone, email, pager, and address info	☐ Yes ☐ No ☐ IP ☐ N/A			
a. Create / maintain a plan to account for all employees during an emergency including the use of recall rosters and conducts quarterly testing of recall rosters	☐ Yes ☐ No ☐ IP ☐ N/A			
12. Establish local network for hospitals and healthcare institutions to monitor and share information during emergencies	☐ Yes ☐ No ☐ IP ☐ N/A			
13. Ensure your Public Health Emergency Officer (PHEO) has attended training and is ready to act in their role during emergencies	☐ Yes ☐ No ☐ IP ☐ N/A			

Hospital Viability Measure:	Compliance IP – In Progress N/A – Not Applicable	Date Initiated	Compliance or Reassessment Date	Actions Required
14. Ensure your Emergency Management Officer has attended training and is assisting in training others in their roles during emergencies	☐ Yes ☐ No ☐ IP ☐ N/A			
15. Ensure your Public Affairs Officer (PAO) is trained to interact with local media and community	☐ Yes ☐ No ☐ IP ☐ N/A			
a. Prepare PAO campaign ahead of time for the hospital during the Pandemic to educate the public about public health measures (Materials may be found at www.cdc.gov/flu/professionals/patiented.htm)	☐ Yes ☐ No ☐ IP ☐ N/A			
16. Ensure staff are pre-fit for PPE and trained on its proper use	☐ Yes ☐ No ☐ IP ☐ N/A			
17. Contract with local manpower pools to provide additional assistance during a pandemic if possible	☐ Yes ☐ No ☐ IP ☐ N/A			
18. Assist local public health department with developing a vaccine distribution plan for implementation 6-9 months after the pandemic started	☐ Yes ☐ No ☐ IP ☐ N/A			
19. Coordinate with State National Guard to plan security and distribution of vaccine when available	☐ Yes ☐ No ☐ IP ☐ N/A			
20. Coordinate with State National Guard to plan for security during distribution of SNS antiviral medications and possible security support at the hospital during the pandemic phase	☐ Yes ☐ No ☐ IP ☐ N/A			

Hospital Viability Measure:	Compliance IP – In Progress N/A – Not Applicable	Date Initiated	Compliance or Reassessment Date	Actions Required
a. Outline procedures for requesting DOD support during emergent situations	☐ Yes ☐ No ☐ IP ☐ N/A			
21. Coordinate with local mortuaries and cemeteries in the development of a mortuary surge plan	☐ Yes ☐ No ☐ IP ☐ N/A			
22. Consider contracting a private security firm to augment existing hospital security during a pandemic	☐ Yes ☐ No ☐ IP ☐ N/A			
23. Document that the following personnel have received training on the facilities influenza plan: Attending Physicians, Environmental Services, Nursing, Lab, ED, Outpatient staff, Security, & Nutrition	☐ Yes ☐ No ☐ IP ☐ N/A			
24. ED staff and Outpatient staff trained in epidemiological monitoring and surveillance in order to familiarize themselves with outbreak trends	☐ Yes ☐ No ☐ IP ☐ N/A			
25. The pandemic response coordinator has contacted local or regional pandemic influenza planning groups to obtain information on communication and coordination plans (For more info on state and local planning visit www.hhs.gov)	☐ Yes ☐ No ☐ IP ☐ N/A			
26. Healthcare facility staff provided with current training opportunities (for example visit www.cdc.gov/flu/professionals/training/ or www/.hhs.gov/pandemicflu/plan/sup4.html)	☐ Yes ☐ No ☐ IP ☐ N/A			

Hospital Viability Measure:	Compliance IP – In Progress N/A – Not Applicable	Date Initiated	Compliance or Reassessment Date	Actions Required
27. Estimates have been made of the quantities of essential patient care materials and equipment such as IV pumps, PPE, pharmaceuticals, and ventilators; that will be needed during an eight-week pandemic with subsequent eight-week pandemic waves	☐ Yes ☐ No ☐ IP ☐ N/A			
28. Develop a list of alternate vendors for medical devices, pharmaceuticals, and contracted services (i.e., laundry, housekeeping, food services)	☐ Yes ☐ No ☐ IP ☐ N/A			
29. Signed agreements have been established with area hospitals and long-term care facilities to accept or receive non-influenza patients who need continued inpatient care	☐ Yes ☐ No ☐ IP ☐ N/A			
30. Create a staffing plan as staffing will be limited during the pandemic phase (up to 40% absenteeism for two weeks during the peak)	☐ Yes ☐ No ☐ IP ☐ N/A			
31. Develop a succession of command roster including delegations of authority	☐ Yes ☐ No ☐ IP ☐ N/A			
32. Review or revise policies on leave, alternative work schedules, and evacuation payments	☐ Yes ☐ No ☐ IP ☐ N/A			
a. Ensure a liberal non-punitive sick leave policy for managing personnel who have symptoms of or documented illness with pandemic influenza	☐ Yes ☐ No ☐ IP ☐ N/A			

Hospital Viability Measure:	Compliance IP – In Progress N/A – Not Applicable	Date Initiated	Compliance or Reassessment Date	Actions Required
b. Policy considers handling of staff who become ill at work and when they may return to work after recovery	☐ Yes ☐ No ☐ IP ☐ N/A			
33. Develop a TELEWORK plan and query staff as to their capabilities at home (i.e., laptops, pre-loaded software, printers, fax, broadband, conference call capability, video teleconference, etc.)	☐ Yes ☐ No ☐ IP ☐ N/A			
34. Determine potential alternative care sites for medical care and plan to operate or supervise them during a pandemic and establish MOU's / contracts (possible sites include schools, gymnasiums, nursing homes, churches, tent hospitals, etc.)	☐ Yes ☐ No ☐ IP ☐ N/A			
35. Develop community-wide childcare options minimizing child overcrowding that would enable staff to continue to work if schools are cancelled	☐ Yes ☐ No ☐ IP ☐ N/A			
36. Develop a set of healthcare roles that may be suitable for volunteers to function during a pandemic and define a protocol for deciding on their suitability for designated roles outside their area of training and competence	☐ Yes ☐ No ☐ IP ☐ N/A			

Hospital Viability Measure:	Compliance IP – In Progress N/A – Not Applicable	Date Initiated	Compliance or Reassessment Date	Actions Required
37. Legal counsel has reviewed up to date emergency laws for employing volunteers with out of state licenses (Consider using a State Emergency System for Advanced Registration of Volunteer Health Professionals ESAR-VHP)	☐ Yes ☐ No ☐ IP ☐ N/A			
38. Legal counsel has reviewed ethical triage plan and concurs with process for providing care with limited resources	☐ Yes ☐ No ☐ IP ☐ N/A			
39. Method in place to rapidly credential providers and nurses assisting with surge consistent with the Joint Commission's disaster privileging standard	☐ Yes ☐ No ☐ IP ☐ N/A			
40. Ensure lab has the capability to test for influenza or maintain multiple contracts for local labs to provide services during the pandemic	☐ Yes ☐ No ☐ IP ☐ N/A			
a. If no lab services are available you may send suspected pandemic influenza samples to: WHO Collaborating Center for Surveillance, Epidemiology and Control of Influenza Centers for Disease Control and Prevention 1600 Clifton Road, Mail Stop G16 Atlanta GA 30333 United States of America Fax: +1 404 639 2334	☐ Yes ☐ No ☐ IP ☐ N/A			

Hospital Viability Measure:	Compliance IP – In Progress N/A – Not Applicable	Date Initiated	Compliance or Reassessment Date	Actions Required
41. Create / review data disaster recovery plan (DRP) annually for securing information technology assets	☐ Yes ☐ No ☐ IP ☐ N/A			
42. Guards have access to lists of emergency numbers for staff, facilities, and IT support available 24 hours a day	☐ Yes ☐ No ☐ IP ☐ N/A			
43. Guards assume front desk duties during heightened threat levels	☐ Yes ☐ No ☐ IP ☐ N/A			
44. Create / maintain an emergency security-staffing plan that includes protocols for staff recall, employee travel, vacation and leave cancellations	☐ Yes ☐ No ☐ IP ☐ N/A			
45. Security Guards receive adequate training to respond to daily operational requirements (DOD facilities must train in accordance with AR 190-56)	☐ Yes ☐ No ☐ IP ☐ N/A			
a. Trained in patient restraint and takedown procedures and authorized to restrain visitors until local law enforcement arrives	☐ Yes ☐ No ☐ IP ☐ N/A			
b. Trained in search/seizure for possible weapons and in the proper administration of handcuffs	☐ Yes ☐ No ☐ IP ☐ N/A			
c. Trained in customer service protocol and techniques and in proper protocol that address handling media and VIP's	☐ Yes ☐ No ☐ IP ☐ N/A			
d. Trained in ―Lock Down" procedures for all or part of the hospital	☐ Yes ☐ No ☐ IP ☐ N/A			

Hospital Viability Measure:	Compliance IP – In Progress N/A – Not Applicable	Date Initiated	Compliance or Reassessment Date	Actions Required
e. Guards are BCLS certified and trained in emergency management roles outlined in HICS	☐ Yes ☐ No ☐ IP ☐ N/A			
Response Phase				
1. Initiate EMP and subsequent emergency plans as soon as CDC or WHO expects epidemic or pandemic	☐ Yes ☐ No ☐ IP ☐ N/A			
2. Initiate PAO campaign plan and educate patients about the hospital's plan and procedures for patients to receive care	☐ Yes ☐ No ☐ IP ☐ N/A			
3. Facilities department ensures signage is present at all entry points including the ED instructing patients and visitors about hospital policies, including notifying staff if they have flu symptoms	☐ Yes ☐ No ☐ IP ☐ N/A			
4. Hospital leadership ensures timely education, training, and risk communication to the staff about the current virus and situation	☐ Yes ☐ No ☐ IP ☐ N/A			
5. Implement rapid training of non-clinical staff to assist with support services: meals, personal care, patient movement, cleaning, etc.	☐ Yes ☐ No ☐ IP ☐ N/A			
6. Ensure staff practice regular hand hygiene often and especially after removing PPE (signs, training, etc,)	☐ Yes ☐ No ☐ IP ☐ N/A			

Hospital Viability Measure:	Compliance IP – In Progress N/A – Not Applicable	Date Initiated	Compliance or Reassessment Date	Actions Required
7. Healthcare workers, patients, and family members are reminded about covering mouth and nose with tissue when coughing or sneezing and perform hand hygiene afterwards (post sign around facility)	☐ Yes ☐ No ☐ IP ☐ N/A			
8. Monitor health of staff exposed to pandemic flu. Antiviral prophylaxis should follow local policy	☐ Yes ☐ No ☐ IP ☐ N/A			
9. Dedicate separate equipment for patients that are suspected or confirmed to have pandemic influenza	☐ Yes ☐ No ☐ IP ☐ N/A			
10. Increase environmental cleaning by disinfecting frequently touched surfaces (i.e. door handles)	☐ Yes ☐ No ☐ IP ☐ N/A			
11. Ensure patient rooms are well ventilated, especially if negative pressure rooms are not available (Opening windows are encouraged)	☐ Yes ☐ No ☐ IP ☐ N/A			
12. Ensure staff use standard and droplet precautions when caring for a patient with and acute, febrile, respiratory illness	☐ Yes ☐ No ☐ IP ☐ N/A			
13. Ensure staff utilize available PPE when treating those with suspected or confirmed pandemic cases	☐ Yes ☐ No ☐ IP ☐ N/A			
a. At a minimum use NIOSH certified N95 surgical or medical mask as part of PPE	☐ Yes ☐ No ☐ IP ☐ N/A			

Hospital Viability Measure:	Compliance IP – In Progress N/A – Not Applicable	Date Initiated	Compliance or Reassessment Date	Actions Required
b. Family members and visitors should practice the same infection control measures and PPE level as hospital staff	☐ Yes ☐ No ☐ IP ☐ N/A			
c. Provide patients with face masks to protect staff and visitors from mucosa of mouth and nose	☐ Yes ☐ No ☐ IP ☐ N/A			
d. Treat any waste that could be contaminated with pandemic virus as infectious clinical waste (i.e. used face masks)	☐ Yes ☐ No ☐ IP ☐ N/A			
14. Limit numbers of staff, family members, or visitors exposed to infected patients	☐ Yes ☐ No ☐ IP ☐ N/A			
15. If possible, avoid overcrowding of patients by providing a single room, or at least 1 meter distance between patients (patients should be arrange head to toe from one another)	☐ Yes ☐ No ☐ IP ☐ N/A			
16. Healthcare staff monitor their own temperatures 2X daily if they have not had the current strain of influenza	☐ Yes ☐ No ☐ IP ☐ N/A			
17. Provide transportation services for staff if needed due to restrictions that may be placed on public transit	☐ Yes ☐ No ☐ IP ☐ N/A			
18. Communicate with and remind employees on how to protect themselves during a pandemic (post signs around the facility)	☐ Yes ☐ No ☐ IP ☐ N/A			

Hospital Viability Measure:	Compliance IP – In Progress N/A – Not Applicable	Date Initiated	Compliance or Reassessment Date	Actions Required
19. Assist local public health department in suggesting rapid action in the implementation of public health measures	☐ Yes ☐ No ☐ IP ☐ N/A			
20. Implement workplace interventions designed to reduce transmission in the workplace such as teleconferences, increased hygiene focus, and working from home if possible	☐ Yes ☐ No ☐ IP ☐ N/A			
21. Assist local government officials, media, and public health to provide honest, helpful, and timely information to the public working to discredit unwarranted fears	☐ Yes ☐ No ☐ IP ☐ N/A			
22. Legal counsel ensures that liability, insurance, and temporary licensing issues for retired healthcare workers and volunteers who may be working outside their training and competence in health and emergency services is within current National practices	☐ Yes ☐ No ☐ IP ☐ N/A			
23. Review and update existing infection control guidelines and consider education needs for healthcare staff, volunteers, and laboratory personnel	☐ Yes ☐ No ☐ IP ☐ N/A			
Response during Pandemic Phase				
1. Defer all non-essential care	☐ Yes ☐ No ☐ IP ☐ N/A			

Hospital Viability Measure:	Compliance IP – In Progress N/A – Not Applicable	Date Initiated	Compliance or Reassessment Date	Actions Required
2. If the patient is stable, discharge to home care with specific influenza discharge recommendations for caregivers including infection control precautions	☐ Yes ☐ No ☐ IP ☐ N/A			
3. Establish 12 hour shifts	☐ Yes ☐ No ☐ IP ☐ N/A			
4. Activate reserve staffing pool	☐ Yes ☐ No ☐ IP ☐ N/A			
5. Establish infected wards to segregate from the rest of the hospital	☐ Yes ☐ No ☐ IP ☐ N/A			
6. increase security presence to ensure a safe environment for patients and employees	☐ Yes ☐ No ☐ IP ☐ N/A			
a. Employ armed security guards at entrance for patient flow and prevent civil disorder	☐ Yes ☐ No ☐ IP ☐ N/A			
b. If possible, limit patients to one entrance in order to control patient access and provide a secure environment	☐ Yes ☐ No ☐ IP ☐ N/A			
c. Enforce hospital access control policies (i.e., issue badges for visitors, patients, and volunteers)	☐ Yes ☐ No ☐ IP ☐ N/A			
d. Maintain a key and essential personnel roster at the entrance allowing access for those who need to respond during the pandemic	☐ Yes ☐ No ☐ IP ☐ N/A			
e. Employ armed security guards at hospital pharmacy to protect medications	☐ Yes ☐ No ☐ IP ☐ N/A			

Hospital Viability Measure:	Compliance IP – In Progress N/A – Not Applicable	Date Initiated	Compliance or Reassessment Date	Actions Required
f. The hospital employs vehicle check points away from the hospital to direct incoming patients and avoid congestion at the entrance	□ Yes □ No □ IP □ N/A			
7. Post staff at entrance to triage and direct patients, hand out face masks if necessary	□ Yes □ No □ IP □ N/A			
a. Designate a specific waiting room for those who have symptoms of PI segregated from other patients	□ Yes □ No □ IP □ N/A			
8. If available, prescribe home healthcare for sub-acute cases	□ Yes □ No □ IP □ N/A			
9. Initiate the Emergency Operations Center (EOC) in the hospital	□ Yes □ No □ IP □ N/A			
a. If possible, create a virtual EOC so staff can work from home and connect through blog sites, chat rooms, phone, teleconference, and email	□ Yes □ No □ IP □ N/A			
b. The EOC should be connected to local, regional, state, and national public health agencies and local responders for surveillance and reporting	□ Yes □ No □ IP □ N/A			
c. Local media should be provided daily updates mixed with public health messages to mitigate some stress on the facility	□ Yes □ No □ IP □ N/A			
Recovery Phase				
1. Employ business continuity plan	□ Yes □ No □ IP □ N/A			

Hospital Viability Measure:	Compliance IP – In Progress N/A – Not Applicable	Date Initiated	Compliance or Reassessment Date	Actions Required
2. Execute existing agreements and operate or supervise care at an alternate care site	☐ Yes ☐ No ☐ IP ☐ N/A			
3. Restock critical logistic supplies during lull in waves of Pandemic	☐ Yes ☐ No ☐ IP ☐ N/A			
4. Transition to case-based surveillance to verify resolution of pandemic wave and to detect emergence of second wave	☐ Yes ☐ No ☐ IP ☐ N/A			
5. Assist local public health in providing information to determine the timeline for rescinding public health mitigation measures	☐ Yes ☐ No ☐ IP ☐ N/A			
6. Conduct After Action Review (AAR) for lessons learned, revise plans	☐ Yes ☐ No ☐ IP ☐ N/A			
7. Define responsibilities for social, psychological and practical support to affected families and companies. If needed, organize training and education for personnel involved	☐ Yes ☐ No ☐ IP ☐ N/A			
8. Assess how existing community groups (religious, volunteer organizations, sports groups, etc.) can contribute to rebuilding the community. Identify contact persons within these groups	☐ Yes ☐ No ☐ IP ☐ N/A			

* Please note, not all items in the checklist will apply to your facility, as the hospital should consider which items are necessary to mitigate identified threats from the Hazard Vulnerability Analysis (HVA). Thus, the not applicable box was added to demonstrate acknowledgement of possible viability measures a facility could utilize. This checklist should help hospital's document compliance with the Joint Commission's Emergency Management standards.

Assessment Conducted by: _____ Date:_____

Signature of CEO:_____ Date:_____

Signature of Hospital Board President or Representative:

_____ Date:_____

Reassessment to be conducted 6 months after the original assessment

Assessment Conducted by: _____ Date:_____

Signature of CEO:_____ Date:_____

Signature of Hospital Board President or Representative:

_____ Date:_____

REFERENCE LIST

American Hospital Association. 2001. ―Chemical and bioterrorism preparedness checklist." *www.aha.org.* October 3. http://www.aha.org/aha/content/ 2001/pdf/MaAt ChecklistB1003.pdf (accessed May 23, 2009).

Association of State and Territorial Health Officials. 2008. ―The strategic national stockpile: Selected promising practices." *www.astho.org.* February. http://www.astho.org/pubs/ASTHOSNSPractices2-08FINAL.pdf (accessed January 26, 2009).

Association of State Correctional Administrators. 2007. ―Preparing the justice system for a pandemic influenza: resources ." *www.ojp.usdoj.gov.* April 16. http://www.ojp.usdoj.gov/BJA/pandemic/ASCAPandemicUpdateVol2.pdf (accessed May 23, 2009).

Avery, George H. et al. 2008. ―Planning for pandemic influenza: Lessons from the experiences of thirteen Indiana vounties." *Journal of Homeland Security and Emergency Management* 5, no. 1: 1-24.

Bardi, Jason S. 2007. ―Rapid response was crucial to containing the 1918 flu pandemic." *www3.niaid.nih.gov.* April 2. http://www3.niaid.nih.gov/news/ newsreleases/ 2007/fluresponse.htm (accessed May 23, 2009).

Barnes, Michael, Carl L Hanson, Len Novilla, Aaron T Meacham, Emily McIntyre, and Brittany C Erickson. 2008. ―Analysis of media agenda setting during and after hurricane Katrina: Implications for emergency preparedness, disaster response, and disaster policy." *American Journal of Public Health* 98, no. 4 (April 2008).

Barry, John M. 2005. *The Great Influenza.* New York: Penquin Group.

Belshe, Robert B. 2005. ―The origins of pandemic influenza - Lessons from the 1918 virus." *The New England Journal of Medicine*, November, 2209-2211.

Blackwell, Jeffery K. 2006. ―Hospital security and force protection: A guide to ensuring patient and employee safety." *www.iroquois.org.* April. http://www.iroquois.org/cmt/cf/documents/Hospital%20Security%20and%20Forc e%20Protection.pdf (accessed May 23, 2009).

Bootsma, Martin C, and Neil M Ferguson. 2007. ―The effect of public health measures on the 1918 influenza pandemic in U.S. cities." *PNAS.* May. 104, no. 18: 7588-7593.

Bowman, Steve, Lawrence Kapp, and Amy Belasco. 2005. ―CRS report for congress hurricane Katrina: DOD disaster response." *www.fas.org.* September 19. http://www.fas.org/sgp/crs/natsec/RL33095.pdf (accessed May 22, 2009).

Brinkerhoff, John R. 2002. ―The posse comitatus act and homeland security.‖ *www.homelandsecurity.org.* February. http://www.homelandsecurity.org/ journal/Articles/brinkerhoffpossecomitatus.htm (accessed October 2, 2008).

Bush, George W. 2003. ―Homeland security presidential directive HSPD-5.‖ *Nimsonline.* February 28. http://www.nimsonline.com/docs/hspd-5.pdf (accessed April 10, 2009).

CA Emergency Medical Services Authority. 2006. ―Hospital incident command system.‖ *CA Emergency Medical Services Authority.* August. http://www.emsa.ca.gov/ HICS/ (accessed January 12, 2009).

Centers for Disease Control and Prevention. 2007. ―Hospital pandemic influenza planning checklist.‖ *www.pandemicflu.gov.* June 1. http://www.pandemicflu.gov/ plan/healthcare/hospitalchecklist.pdf (accessed May 23, 2009).

———. 2009. ―Interim CDC guidance for nonpharmaceutical community mitigation in response to human infections with swine influenza (H1N1) virus.‖ *www.iaam.org.* April 28. http://www.iaam.org/CVMS/Non-Pharmaceutical.pdf (accessed May 23, 2009).

———. 2009. ―Interim guidance for infection control for care of patients with confirmed or suspected swine influenza A (H1N1) virus infection in a healthcare setting.‖ *www.cdc.gov.* April 29. http://www.cdc.gov/h1n1flu/ guidelines_infection_control.htm (accessed May 23, 2009).

———. 2007. ―Interim pre-pandemic planning guidance: community strategy for pandemic influenza mitigation in the United States.‖ *www.healthvermont.gov.* February. http://healthvermont.gov/panflu/documents/0207interimguidance.pdf (accessed May 23, 2009).

———. 2005. ―State and local pandemic influenza planning checklist.‖ *www.pandemicflu.gov.* December 2. http://www.pandemicflu.gov/plan/states/ statelocalchecklist.html (accessed May 23, 2009).

Central Intelligence Agency. 2003. ―SARS lessons from the first epidemic of the 21st century a collaborative analysis with outside experts (U).‖ *www.nie.wikispaces.com.* September 29. http://nie.wikispaces.com/ SARS++Lessons+From+the+First+Epidemic+of+the+21st+Century+A+Collabor ative+Analysis+With+Outside+Experts+(U) (accessed May 23, 2009).

Communicable Disease Epidemiology Section. 2008. ―Triggers and actions for influenza pandemic response in wisconsin.‖ *http://pandemic.wisconsin.gov.* July 15. http://pandemic.wisconsin.gov/section.asp?linkid=1208&locid=106 (accessed May 22, 2009).

Cretikos, Michelle et al. 2008. "Household disaster preparedness and information sources: Rapid cluster survy after a storm in New South Wales, Australia." *BMC Public Health.*

Davenport, R. John. 2008. "The next pandemic: Bird flu and the 1918 scourge yield harbingers of threats to come." *www.infection-research.de.* June 17. http://www.infection-research.de/perspectives/detail/pressrelease/the_next_pandemic_bird_flu_and_the_1918_scourge_yield_harbingers_of_threats_to_come/ (accessed May 21, 2009).

Dayton, Christopher et al. 2008. "Integrated plan to augment surge capacity." *Prehospital and Disaster Medicine* 23, no. 2 (March-April): 113-120.

Draper, Healther et al. 2008. "Healthcare workers' attitudes towards working during pandemic influenza: A multi method study." *BMC Public Health.*

Ehrenstein, Boris P, Frank Hanses, and Bernd Salzberger. 2006. "Influenza pandemic and professional duty: Family or patients first? A survey of hospital employees." *BMC Public Health,* December.

Emergency Medical Services Authority. 2006. "Disaster medical services division — hospital incident command system (HICS) FAQ's." *www.emsa.ca.gov.* October. http://www.emsa.ca.gov/HICS/default.asp (accessed May 19, 2009).

Engman, Martin L. 2002. "SARS Outbreak and Lessons Learned." *Journal of Insurance Medicine.* 83-85.

Federal Financial Institutions Examination Council. 2009. "Lessons Learned From Hurricane Katrina." *www.ffiec.gov.* March 23. http://www.ffiec.gov/katrina_lessons.htm (accessed May 23, 2009).

Food Marketing Institute. 2006. "Food Safety and Defense." *Food Marketing Institute.* March. http://www.fmi.org/foodsafety/?fuseaction=avian_flu (accessed March 19, 2009).

Government Accounting Office. 2003. "Hospital Preparedness: Most Urban Hospital Have Emergency Plans but Lack Certain Capacities for Bioterrorism Response."

———. 2005. "Hurricane Katrina: Providing oversight of the nation's preparedness, response, and recovery activities." *www.gao.gov.* September 28. http://www.gao.gov/new.items/d051053t.pdf (accessed 05 22, 2009).

Garcia-Sastre, Adolfo, and Richard J. Whitley. 2006. "Lessons learned from reconstructing the 1918 influenza pandemic." *The Journal of Infectious Diseases.* 127-132.

Garrett, Thomas A. 2008. "Pandemic economics: The 1918 influenza and its modern-day implications." *Federal Reserve Bank of St. Louis Review* 90, no. 2 (March / April): 75-93.

Glabman, Maureen. 2001. "Bioterrorism: The silent killer." *Trustee*, November/December. 29-33.

Gonzalez, Jesse C. 2002. "Delivering security in today's new threat environments." *Journal of Healthcare Protection Management* 18, 35-38.

Haque, Azizul, Didier Hober, and Lloyd Kaspert. 2007. "Confronting potential influenza A (H5N1) pandemic with better vaccines." *Emerging Infectious Diseases* 13, no. 10 (October): 1512-1518.

Hatchett, Richard J, Carter E Mecher, and Marc Lipstich. 2007. "Public health interventions and epidemic intensity during the 1918 pandemic." *PNAS* 104, no. 18 (May): 7582-7587.

Henning, Kelly J, Patrick J Brennan, Cindy Hoegg, Eileen O'Rourke, Bernard D Dyer, and Thomas L Grace. 2004. "Health system preparedness for bioterrorism: Bringing the tabletop to the hospital." *Infection Control And Hospital Epidemiology* 25, no. 2 (February): 146-155.

Horton, Kevin D, Maureen Orr, Theodora Tsongas, Richard Leiker, and Vikas Kapil. 2008. "Secondary contamination of medical personnel, equipment, and facilities resulting from hazardous materials events, 2003-2006." *Disaster Medicine and Public Health Preparedness* 2, no. 2. 104-113.

Indiana State Department of Health. 2006. "Pandemic influenza plan." *www.in.gov.* October. http://www.in.gov/isdh/files/PandemicInfluenzaPlan.pdf (accessed January 26, 2009).

———. "Pandemic influenza plan." 2006. *www.in.gov.* October. http://www.in.gov/isdh/files/PandemicInfluenzaPlan.pdf (accessed May 23, 2009).

Kelman, Ilan. 2008. "Lessons relearned from Katrina?" *American Journal of Disaster Medicine* 3, no. 2 (March / April): 61-62.

Kilbourne, Edwin D. 2006. "Influenza Pandemics of the 20th Century." *Emerging Infectious Diseases* 12, no. 1 (January): 9-14.

Lazzari, Stephano, and Klaus Stohr. 2004. "Avian influenza and influenza pandemics." *Bulletin of the World Health Organization*, April. 242.

Lessons Learned Information Sharing. Nd. "Harris County, Texas Citizen Corps' response to Hurricane Katrina." *www.citizencorps.gov.*

https://www.citizencorps.gov/pdf/llis/lessons-learned-tx-katrina-response.pdf (accessed May 22, 2009).

Lister, Sarah A. 2005. ―Pandemic influenza: Domestic preparedness efforts.‖ *www.fas.org.* November 10. http://www.fas.org/sgp/crs/homesec/RL33145.pdf (accessed May 23, 2009).

Luke, Thomas C, and Jean-Paul Rodrigue. 2008. ―Protecting public health and global freight transportation systems during an influenza pandemic.‖ *American Journal of Disaster Medicine* 3: 99-107.

Macey, Jeannette, Theresa Tam, and Arlene King. 2005 ―Public health strategies SARS in Canada.‖ *www.portal.saude.gov.* November 16. http://portal.saude.gov.br/ portal/arquivos/pdf/jeannete_macey3.pdf (accessed May 23, 2009).

Madrid, Paula A, and Roy Grant. 2008. ―Meeting mental health needs following a natural disaster: Lessons from hurricane Katrina.‖ *Professional Psychology: Research and Practice.* 86-91.

Mahoney, Patrick. 2008. ―1918 influenza pandemic: Lessons for homeland security.‖ *Fire Engineering* 161, no. 7 (July): 111-114.

McGlown, K. Joanne, ed. 2004. *Terrorism and Disaster Management.* Chicago, IL, IL: Health Administration Press.

Nevada Hospital Association. 2007. ―Evolution of the Joint Commission Emergency Management Standards.‖ *Nevada Hospital Association.* http://www.nvha.net/ bio/postings/jcstandards.pdf (accessed May 13, 2009).

——.2008. ―Hospital preparedness for tomorrow's healthcare challenges.‖ *Nevada Hospital Association.* http://www.nvha.net/bio/postings/jcstandards.pdf (accessed May 12, 2009).

——. Nd. ―Hospital-based mass prophylaxis and vaccination strategy.‖ Nevada: Nevada Hospital Association.

Nuno, M, T. A Reichert, G Chowell, and A. B Gumel. 2008. ―Protecting residentail care facilities from pandemic influenza.‖ Edited by Simon A Levin. *PNAS* 105, no. 30 (July): 10625-10630.

O'Boyle, Carol, Cheryl Robertson, and Molly Secor-Turner. 2006. ―Nurses' beliefs about public health emergencies: Fear of abandonment.‖ *American Journal of Infection Control* 34, no. 6. 351-357.

OSHA. 2007. ―Guidance on preparing workplaces for an influenza pandemic.‖ *www.OSHA.gov.* http://www.osha.gov/Publications/OSHA3327pandemic.pdf (accessed October 15, 2008).

Penhaul, Karl. 2009. ―Swine flu fears stalk the living and the dead in Mexico City." *CNN News.* May 1. http://edition.cnn.com/2009/WORLD/americas/05/01/ penhaul.mexico.flu/ (accessed May 13, 2009).

Pietrzak, Michael P. 2004. ―Threat mitigation in hospital design." *Hospital Engineering & Facilities Management.*

Ransom, Montrece McNeill, Richard A Goodman, and Anthony D Moulton. 2008. ―Addressing gaps in health care sector legal preparedness for public health emergencies." *Disaster Medicine and Public Health Preparedness* 2, no. 1, 50-56.

Rothstein, Mark et al. 2003. ―Quarantine and isolation: Lessons learned from SARS." *www.iaclea.org.* November 2003. http://www.iaclea.org/members/pdfs/ SARS%20REPORT.Rothstein.pdf (accessed May 23, 2009).

Scahill, Jeremy. 2005. *Blackwater Down.* September 22.

Scheips, Paul J. 2005. *The Role of Federal Military Forces in Domestic Disorders 1945-1992.* Washington D.C.: Center of Military History.

Schoch-Spana, Monica. 2000. ―Implications of pandemic influenza for bioterrorism response." Edited by Donald A Henderson, Thomas V Jr. Inglesby and Tara O'Toole. *Clinical Infectious Diseases*, December: 1409-1413.

Siegel, Judy. 2006. ―US healthcare workers not ready for flu pandemic. Israeli-aided study shows 40% wouldn't report to work." *Jerusalem Post*, April 21, 2006: 8.

SMT Security. 2008. *SMT Security.* http://www.smtsecurity.com/ (accessed October 22, 2008).

Steinhauer, Rene, and Jeff Bauer. 2002. ―The emergency management plan." *RN* 65, no. 6 (June): 40-46.

Svoboda, Tomislav et al. 2004. ―Public health measures to control the spread of the severe acute respiratory syndrome during the outbreak in Toronto." *The New England Journal of Medicine* 350, no. 23 (June): 2352-2361.

Tabery, J, and Charles W Mackett III. 2008. ―Ethics of Triage in the Event of an Influenza Pandemic." *Disaster Medicine and Public Health Preparedness* 2, no. 2, 114-118.

The Institute for Crisis, Disaster, and Risk Management (ICDRM) at the George Washington University (GWU); for the Veterans Health Administration. 2006. ―Emergency management principles and practices for healthcare systems." *Veterans Affairs.* June. http://www1.va.gov/emshg/docs/EMA_Unit1_ Emergency_Management_Programs.pdf (accessed October 23, 2008).

The Joint Commission. 2008. "The Joint Commission accreditation program: Hospital emergency management." *www.jointcommission.org.* 2008. http://www.jointcommission.org/ (accessed Oct 15, 2008).

The National Response Team. 2000. "Incident command system/unified command (ICS/UC)." *www.nrt.org.* http://www.nrt.org/Production/NRT/NRTWeb.nsf/ AllAttachmentsByTitle/SA-52ICSUCTA/$File/ICSUCTA.pdf?OpenElement (accessed May 19, 2009).

Thompson, Nancy A, and Christopher D Van Gorder. 2007. "Healthcare executives' role in preparing for the pandemic influenza 'gap': A new paradigm for disaster planning?" *Journal of Healthcare Management* 52, no. 2 (Mar/Apr): 87-93.

Toner, Eric et al. 2006. "Hospital preparedness for pandemic influenza." *Biosecurity and Bioterrorism* 4, no. 2 (June): 207-217.

U.S. Department of Defense. 2004. "Department of Defense guidance for preparation and response to an influenza pandemic cause by the bird flu (avian influenza)." *DOD Geis web.* Septemeber 21. http://www.geis.fhp.osd.mil/GEIS/ SurveillanceActivities/Influenza/DoD_Flu_Plan_040921.pdf (accessed January 26, 2009).

———2006. "DOD implementation plan for pandemic influenza." *www.fhp.osd.mil.* 08. http://fhp.osd.mil/aiWatchboard/pdf/DoD_PI_Implementation_Plan_August_200 6_Public_Release.pdf (accessed 05 13, 2009).

———2006. "The Federal Response to Hurricane Katrina Lessons Learned." *http://georgewbush-whitehouse.archives.gov.* February. http://georgewbush-whitehouse.archives.gov/reports/katrina-lessons-learned/ (accessed May 22, 2009).

U.S. Department of Health Affairs. 2006. "HA policies." *Military Health System.* Edited by David Chu. January 10, 2006. http://www.health.mil/ hapolicies.aspx?policyYear=2006 (accessed March 4, 2009).

U.S. Department of Health and Human Services. 2008. "Key elements of departmental pandemic influenza operational plans." *www.pandemicflu.gov.* August. http://www.pandemicflu.gov/plan/federal/operationalplans.html (accessed May 23, 2009).

———2005. "HHS pandemic influenza plan." *www.bvsde.paho.org.* November. http://www.bvsde.paho.org/bvsacd/cd63/HHSPandemic/conten.pdf (accessed May 23, 2009).

U.S. Department of Homeland Security. 2008. "National incident command system." *www.fema.gov.* December. http://www.fema.gov/pdf/emergency/nims/ NIMS_core.pdf (accessed 05 19, 2009).

————2004. ―National incident management system." *Department of Homeland security.* March 1. http://www.nimsonline.com/ (accessed January 12, 2009).

————2006. ―National strategy for pandemic influenza implementation plan." *Whitehouse.gov.* May. http://www.whitehouse.gov/homeland/pandemic-influenza-implementation.html (accessed January 12, 2009).

————2006. ―Pandemic influenza, preparedness, response, and recovery guide for critical infrastructure and key resources." *Department of Homeland Security.* September 19. http://www.ready.gov/business/_downloads/ pandemic_influenza.pdf (accessed January 12, 2009).

United States Code. 1878. *Posse Comitatus Act.* June 18.

US Department of Health and Human Services. Nd. ―Take the lead: Working together to prepare now." *pandemicflu.gov.* http://www.pandemicflu.gov/takethelead/ fact_sheet_basics.pdf (accessed September 22, 2008).

Wong, Teck Yee et al. 2008. ―A cross-sectional study of primary-care physicians in Singapore on their concerns and preparedness for an avian influenza outbreak." *Annals Academy of Medicine*, 458-464.

World Health Organization. 2009 ―Infection prevention and control in health care in providing care for confirmed or suspected A(H1N1) swine influenza patients." *www.who.int.* April 29. www.who.int/entity/csr/resources/publications /20090429_infection_control_en.pdf (accessed May 23, 2009).

————2009. ―Pandemic influenza preparedness and response." *www.who.int.* April. www.who.int/entity/csr/disease/influenza/PIPGuidance09.pdf (accessed May 1, 2009).

————2008. ―Excess mortality rates from common illnesses during an influenza reducing pandemic." *www.who.int.* http://www.who.int/csr/resources/ publications/swineflu/commonillnesses_pandemic/en/index.html (accessed May 23, 2009).

————2003. ―SARS: Status of the outbreak and lessons for the immediate future." *www.who.int.* May 20. http://www.who.int/csr/media/sars_wha.pdf (accessed May 23, 2009).

————2005. ―WHO Checklist for Influenza Pandemic Preparedness Planning." *www.who.int.* http://www.who.int/csr/resources/publications/influenza/ WHO_CDS_CSR_GIP_2005_4/en/ (accessed May 23, 2009).

Yale New Haven Health. Nd. ―Pandemic influenza hospital preparedness checklist." *www.yalenewhavenhealth.org.* http://yalenewhavenhealth.org/emergency/ commu/Pandemic_flu_hospital_checklist.pdf (accessed May 23, 2009).